The Ultimate Stretching Manual

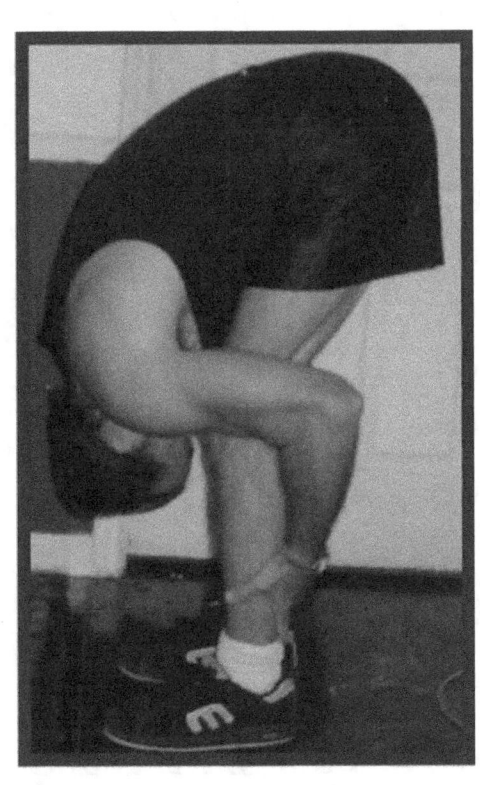

Shoulder Stretches

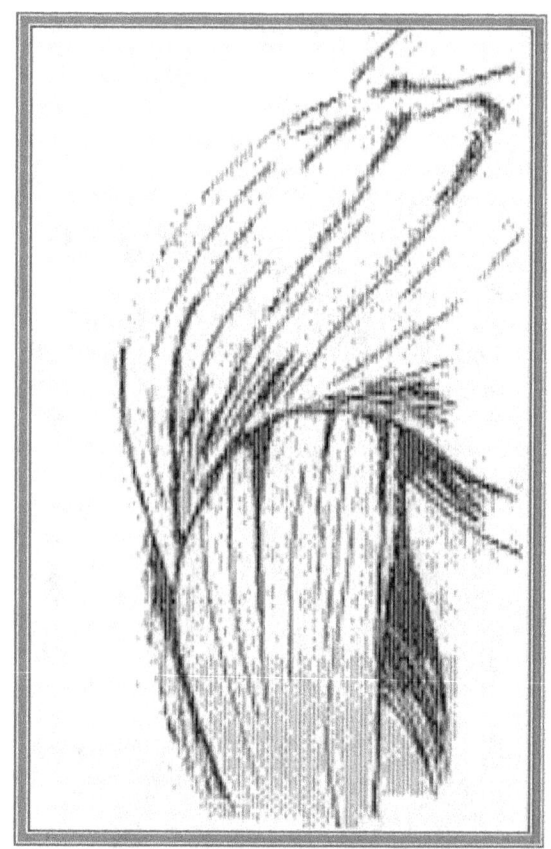

Do all stretches 6 to 8 times. Relax and breath easy, do not bounce or force the stretch..

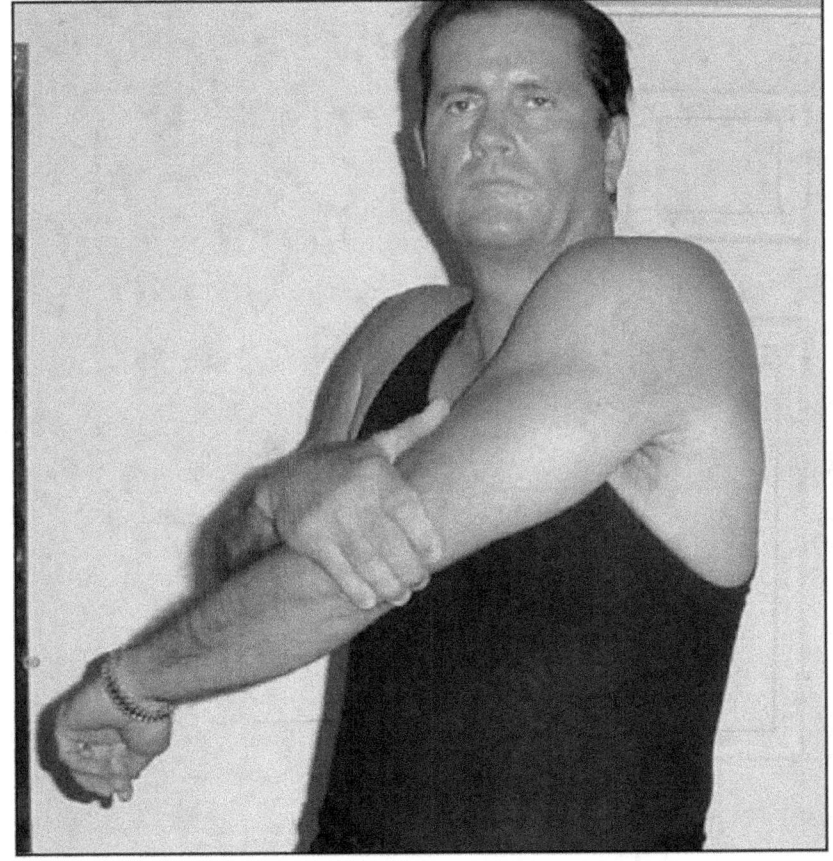

Reach across the body and grab the elbow. Pull it gently across your body.

Reach behind your body and grab the wrist of one arm, gently pull the wrist behind your back.

While holding your wrist with the other arm lean forward to stretch. Repeat to both sides.

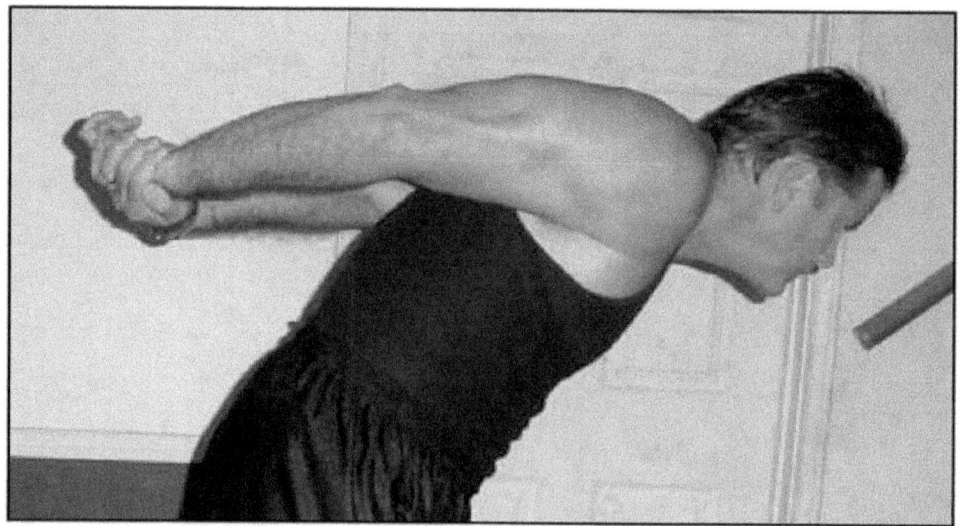

Here we are doing arm circles. Hold the hands pointed to the sides and make large gentle swings of the arms around the body.

Shrug the shoulders forward and backwards to loosen them.

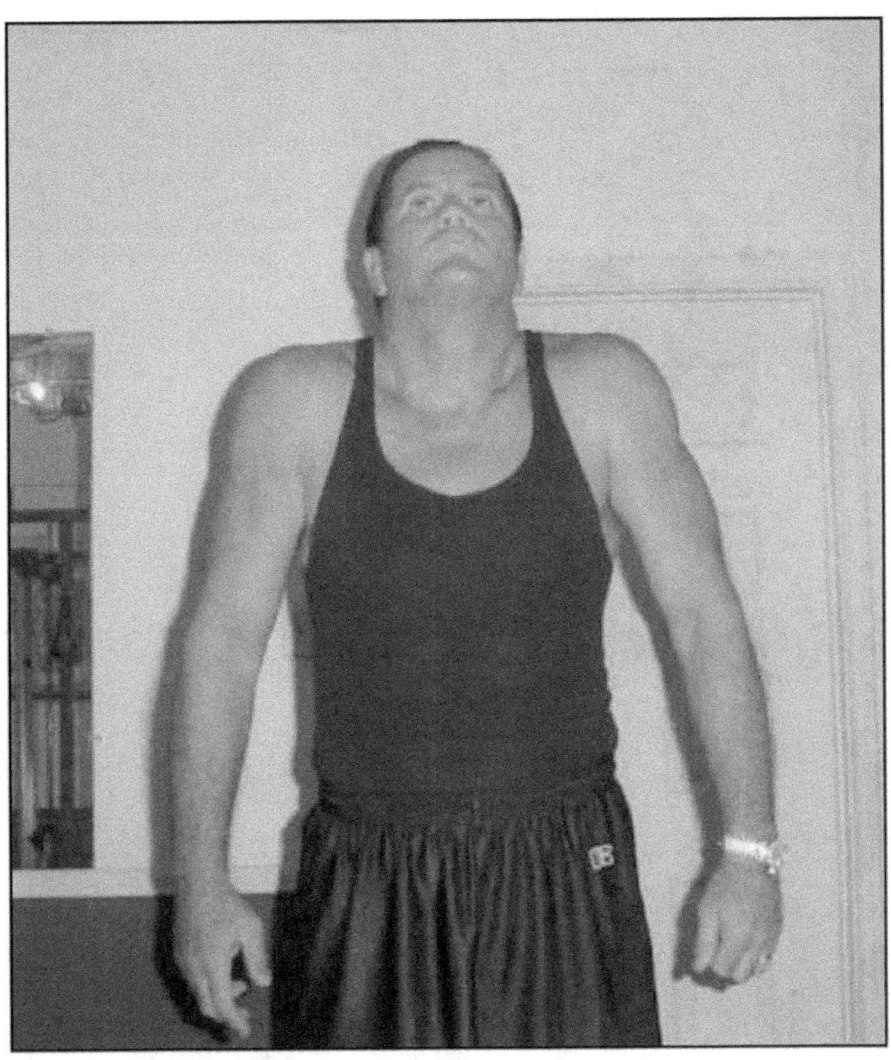

Here we do a modified arm swing. Hold the arms straight to the sides and swing them up as high as possible to the front.

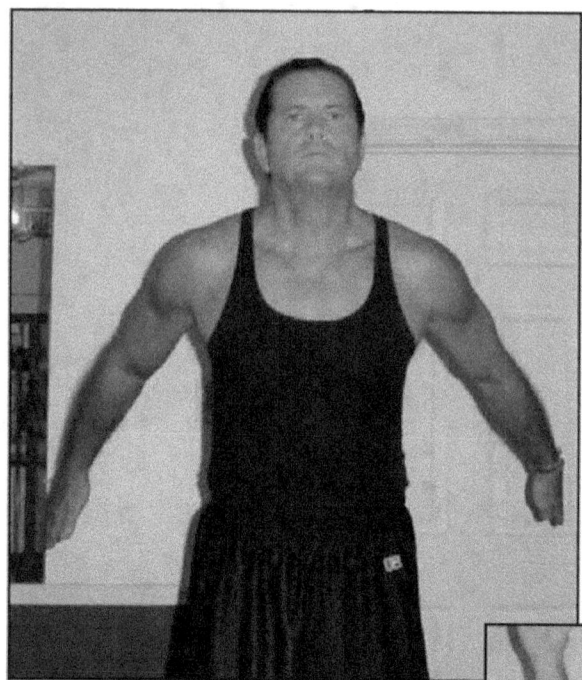

Here we do a modified arm swing. Hold the arms straight to the sides and swing them up as high as possible to the front.

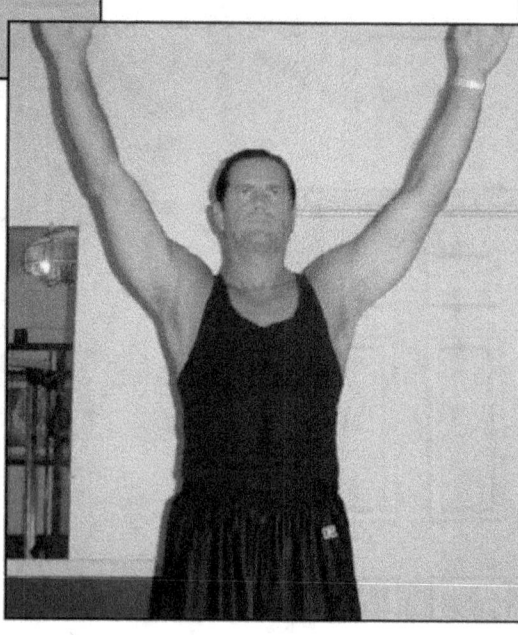

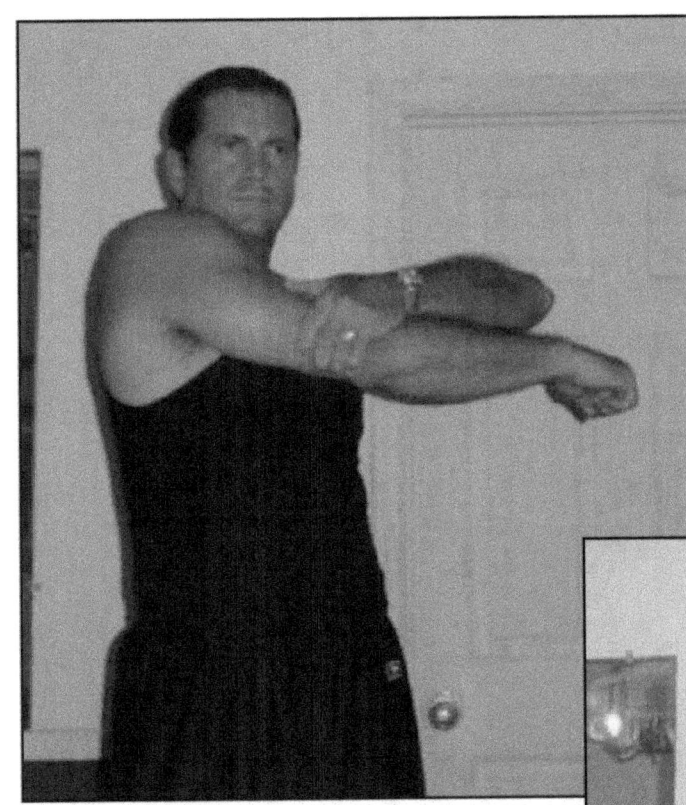

Reach up and grab the tricep of the opposite arm and pull it across the body.

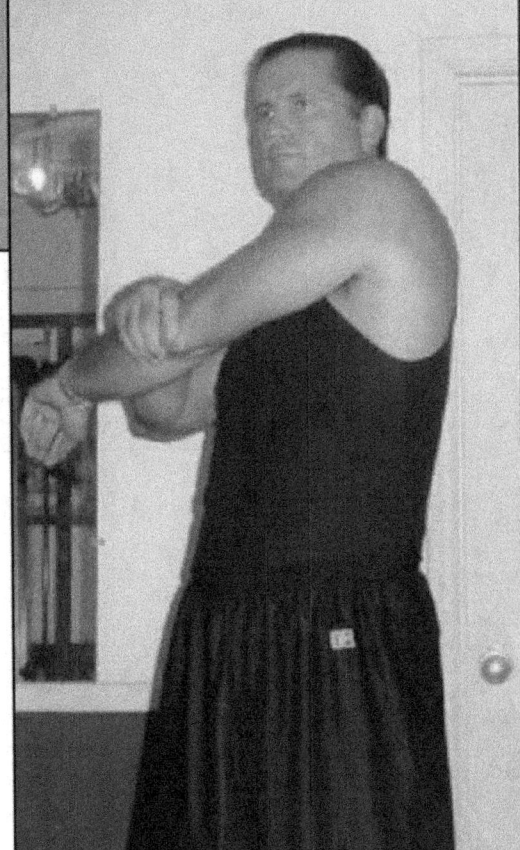

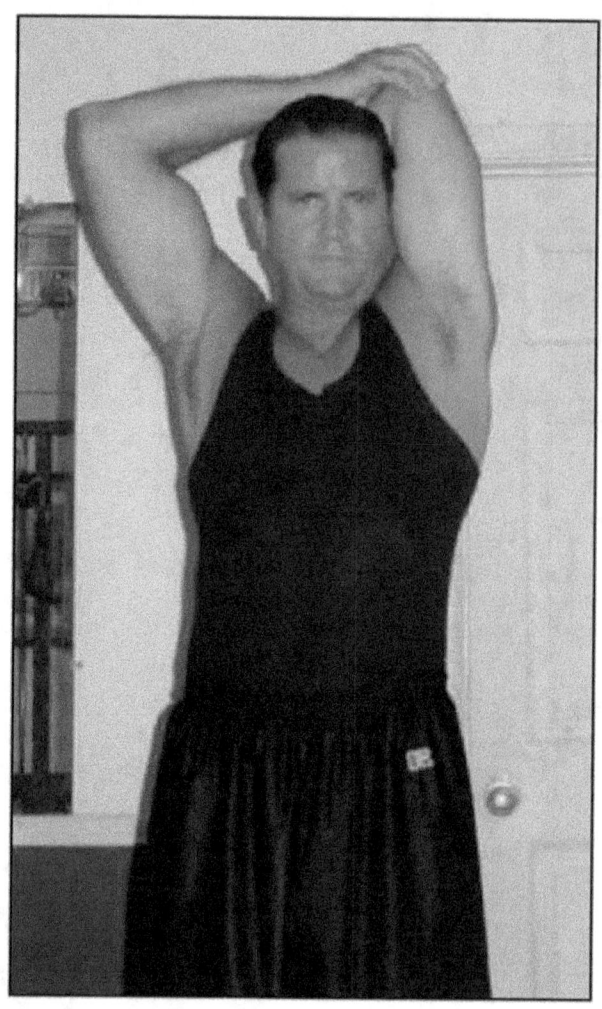

Reach up and grab the tricep of the opposite arm and pull it across the body.

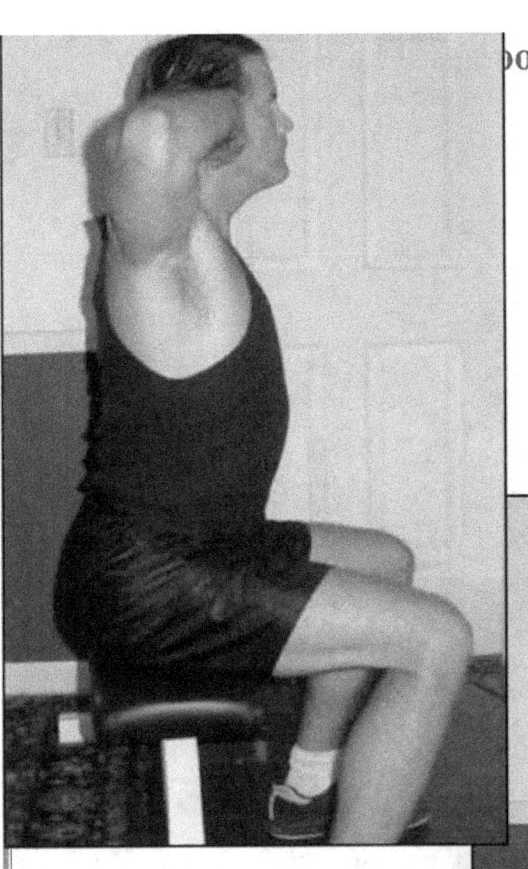

Place the arms on the back of the neck and flex them to stretch the chest and shoulders.

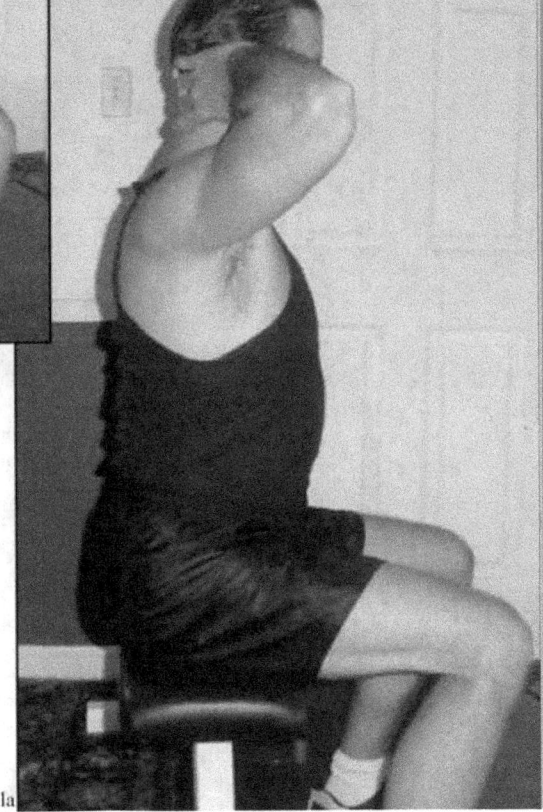

Reach out and hold the wall
while pulling the body
forward.

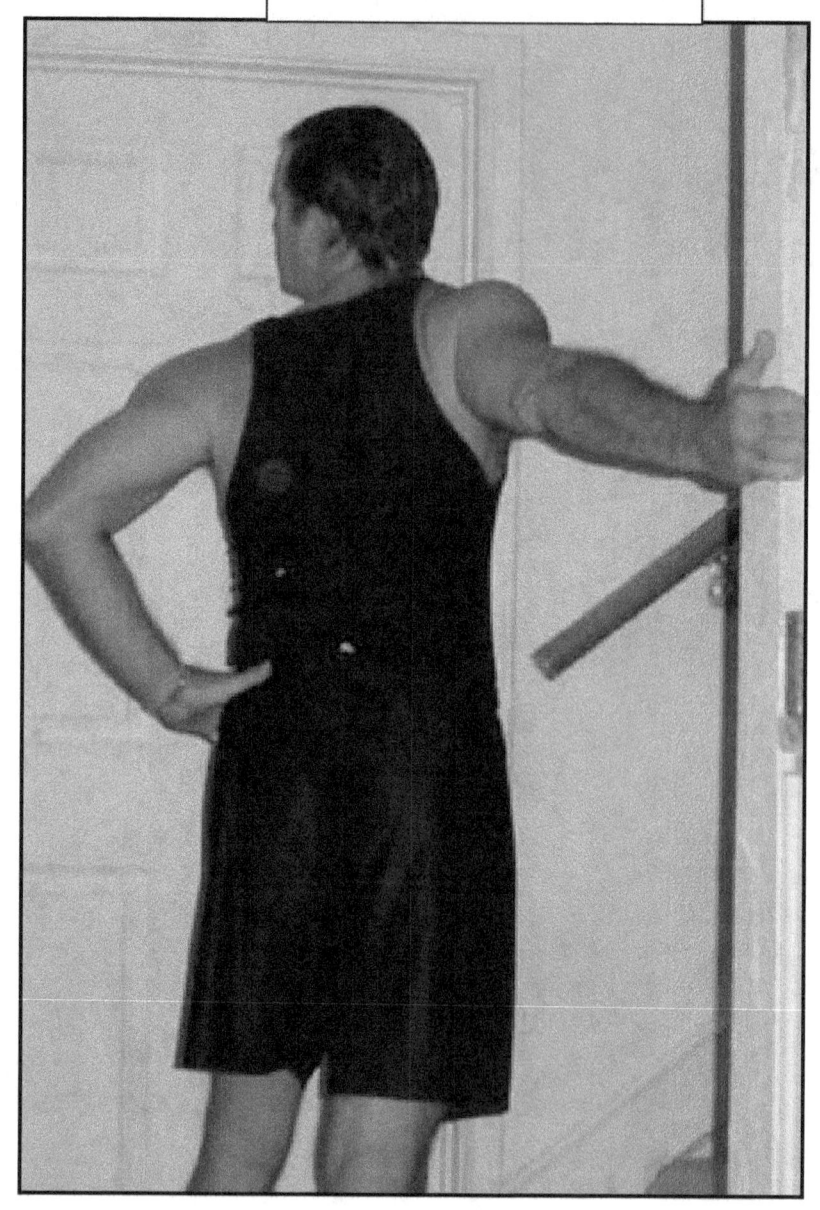

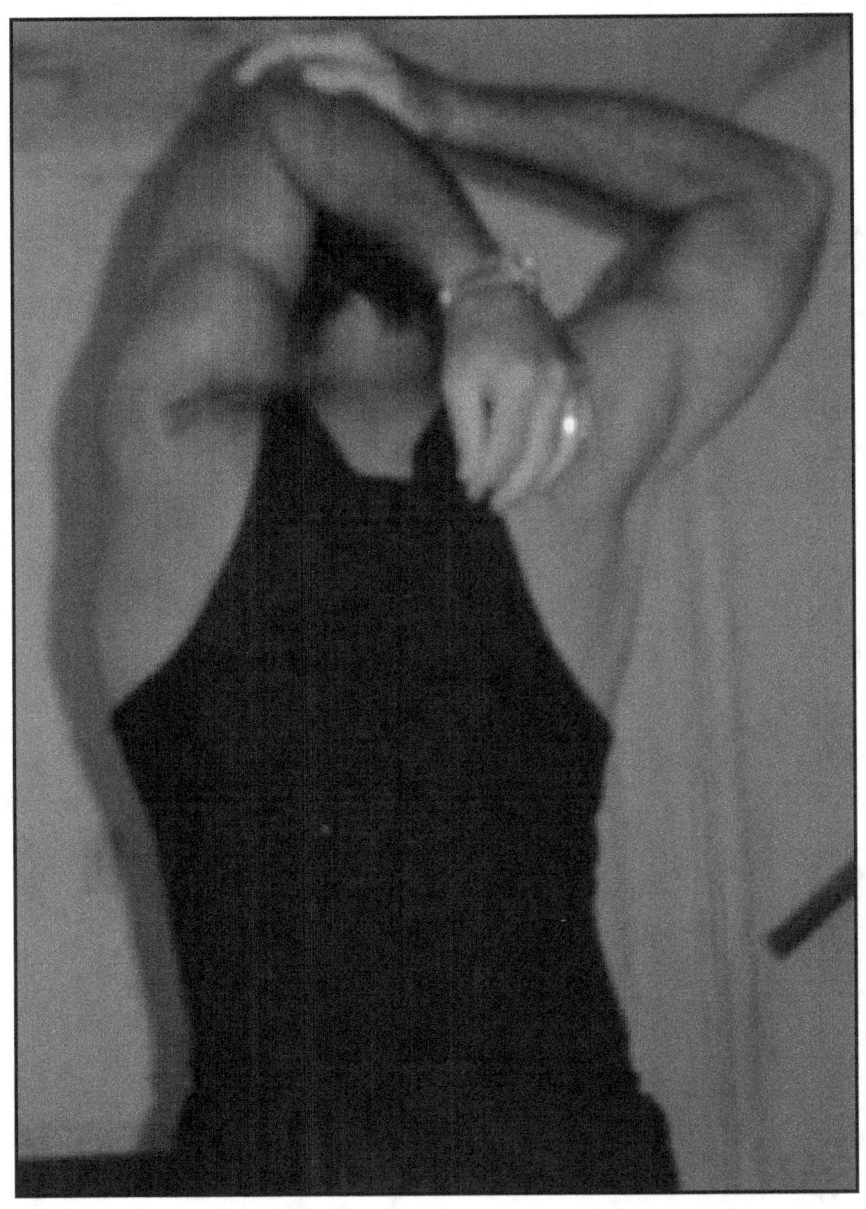

Reach up and grab the tricep of the opposite arm and pull it down across the back.

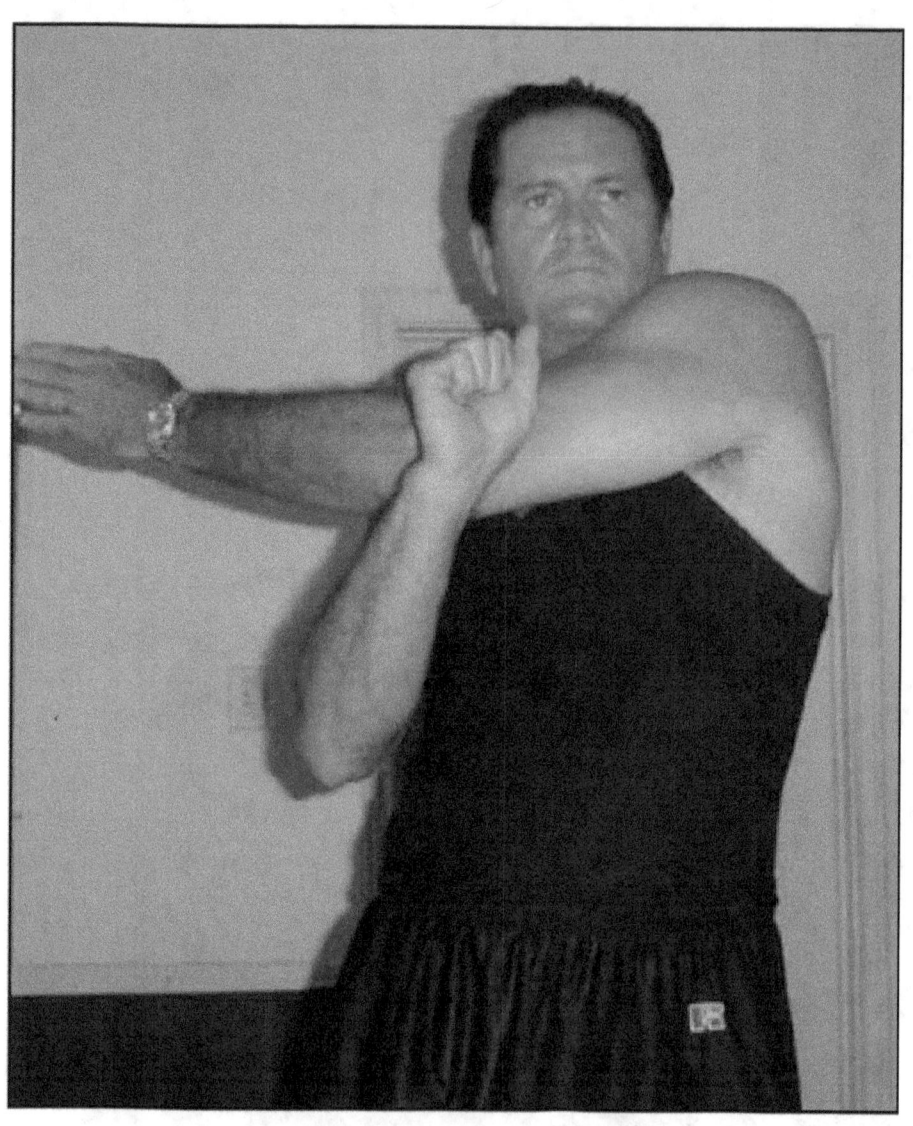

Reach up and grab the tricep of the opposite arm and pull it across the body.

Lean back against the bar and drop the body down as if doing a reverse dip. Use the legs for support.

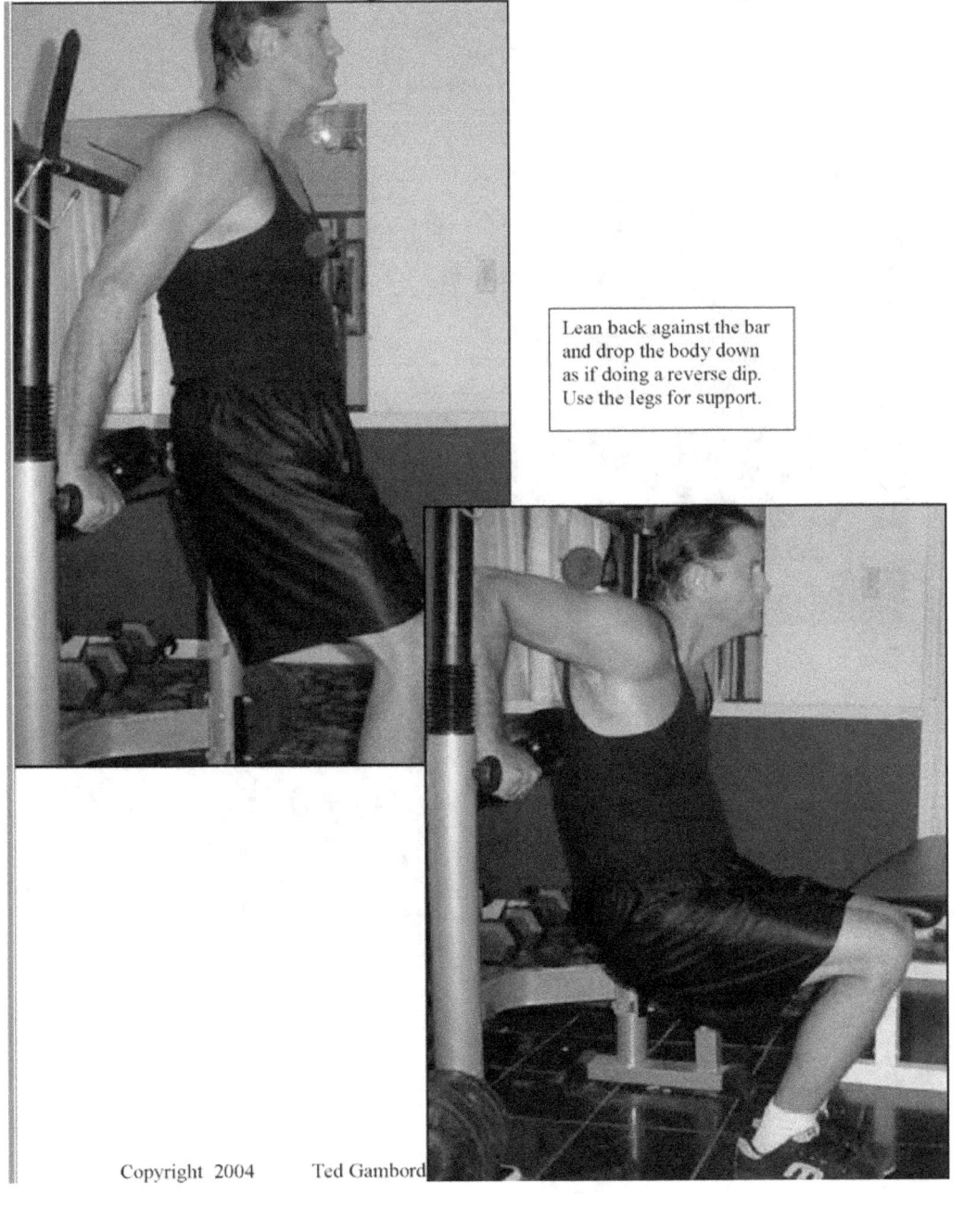

Lean back against the bar
and drop the body down
as if doing a reverse dip.
Use the legs for support.

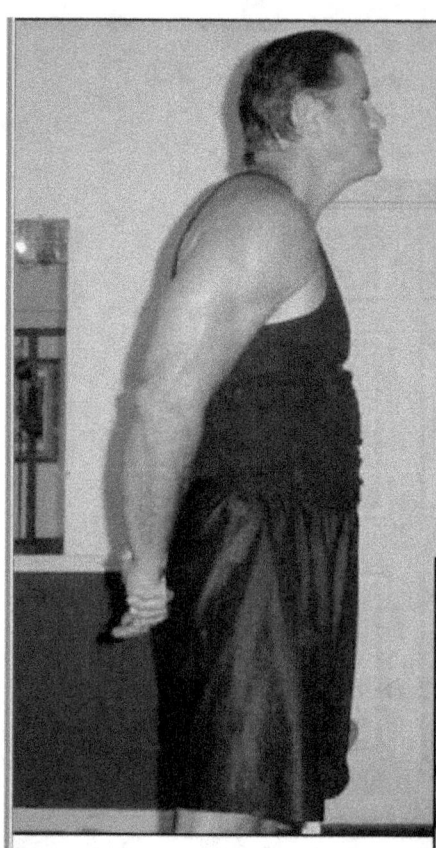

Reach around and grab the
wrist of one arm with the
other, then lean forward
and stretch it.

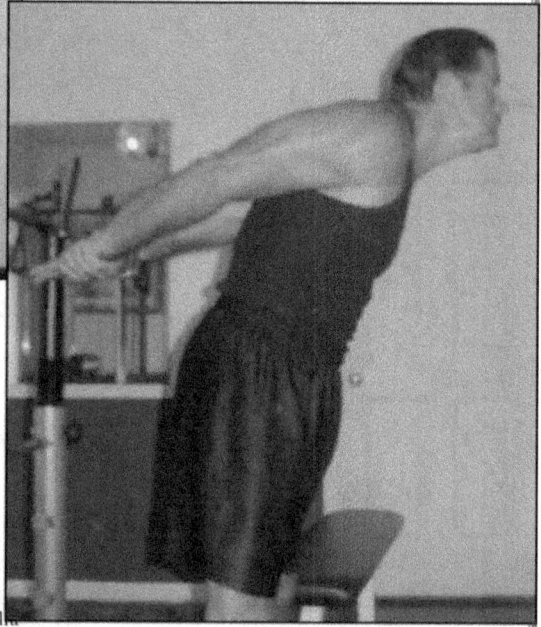

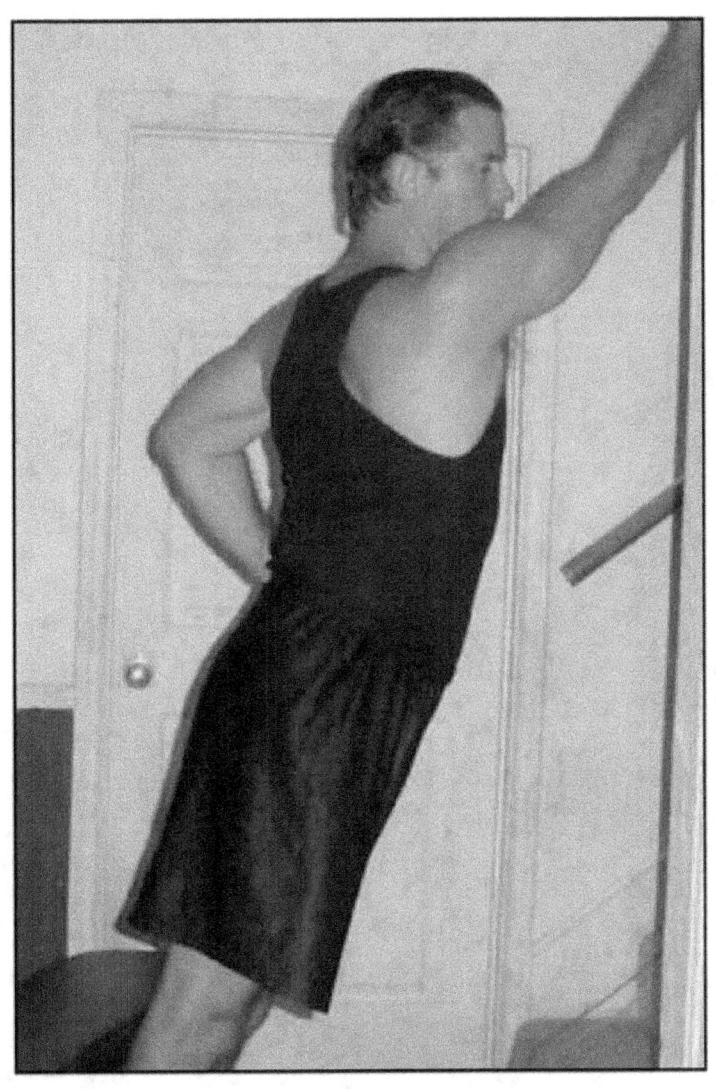

Lean out to the wall and hold one arm on the wall and you stretch forward.

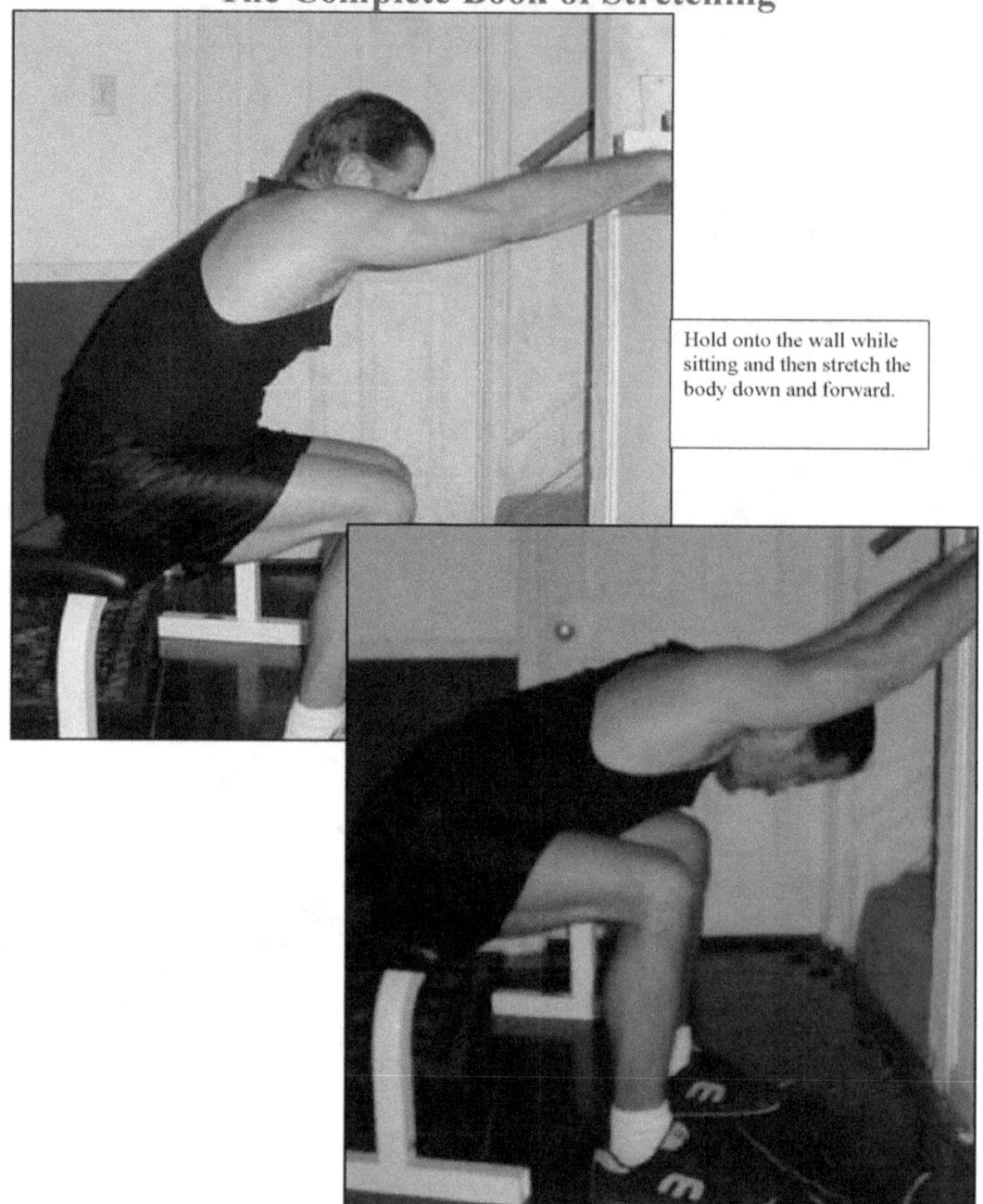

Hold onto the wall while sitting and then stretch the body down and forward.

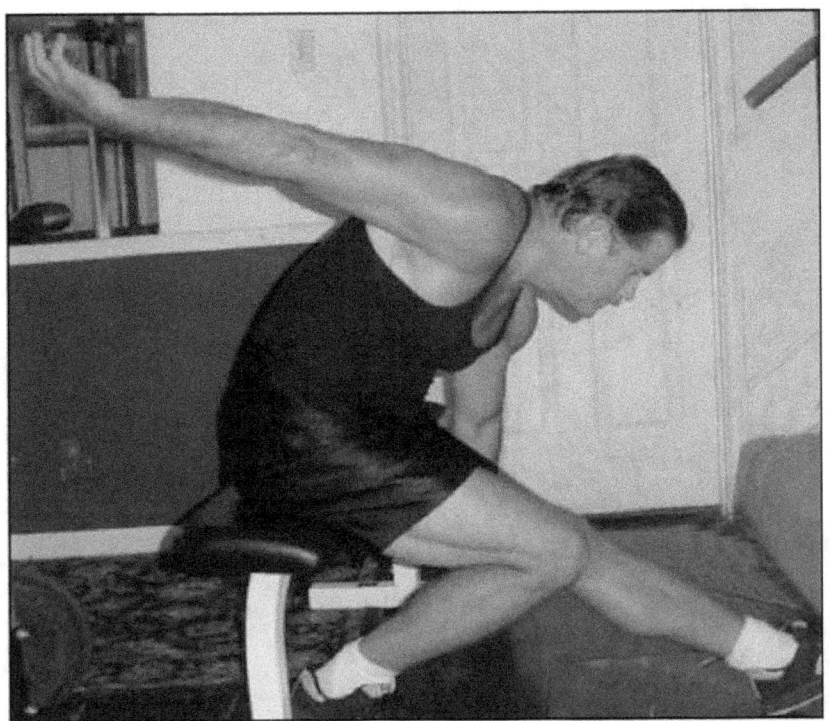

Put one leg straight out while sitting and reach back with the opposite arm. Alternate arms.

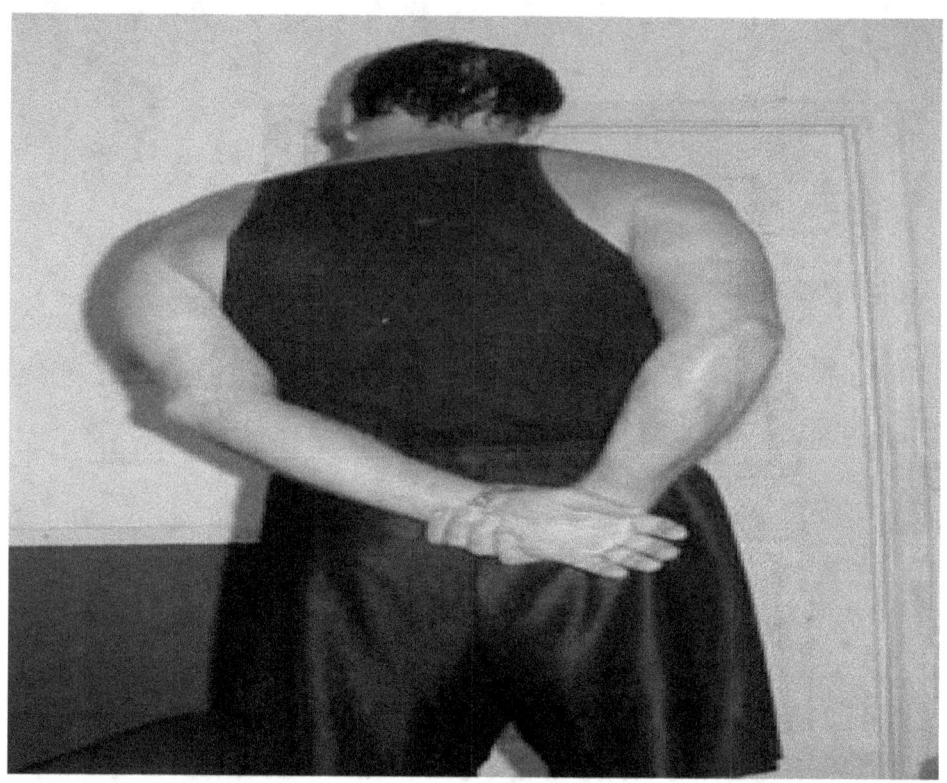

Reach back and grab the wrist and pull the arm across the back of the body.

Reach up and grab the tricep of the opposite arm and lift it up as far as possible towards the back

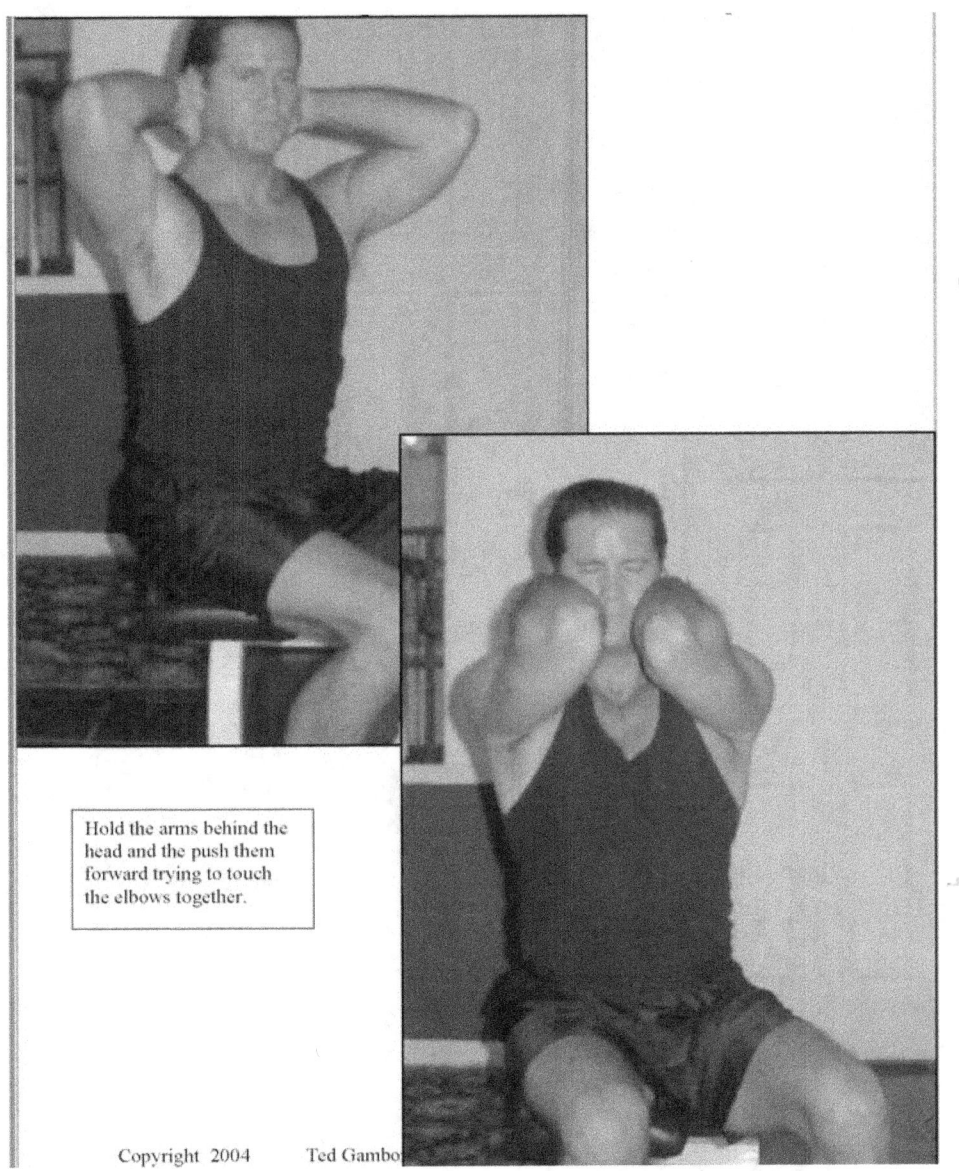

Hold the arms behind the head and the push them forward trying to touch the elbows together.

Copyright 2004 Ted Gambo

Hold the arms behind the head and the push them forward trying to touch the elbows together.

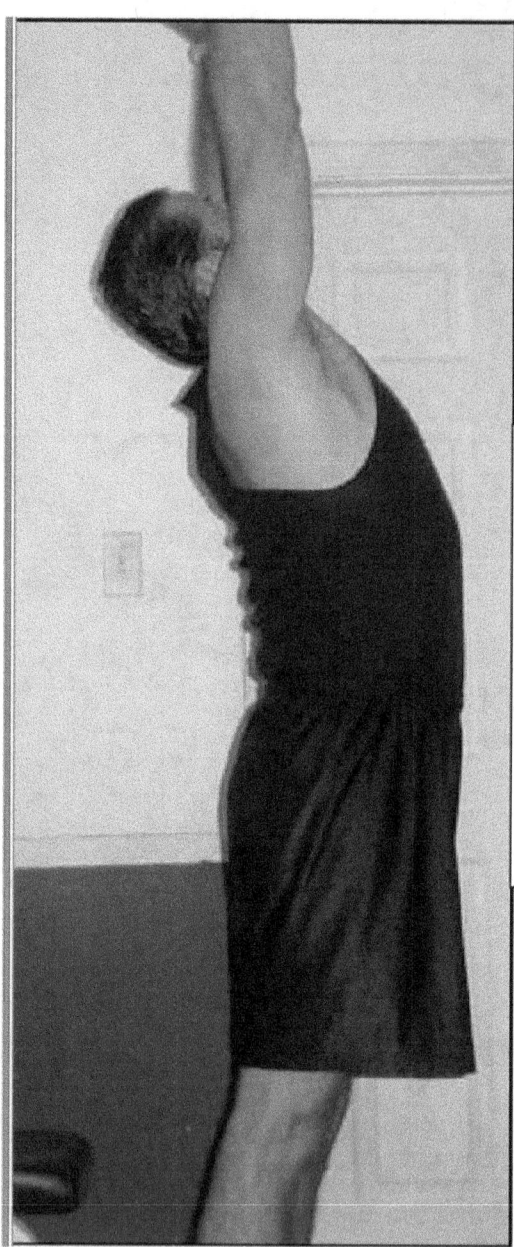

Stand very tall and reach up, then stretch up to the toes while reaching as high as you can.

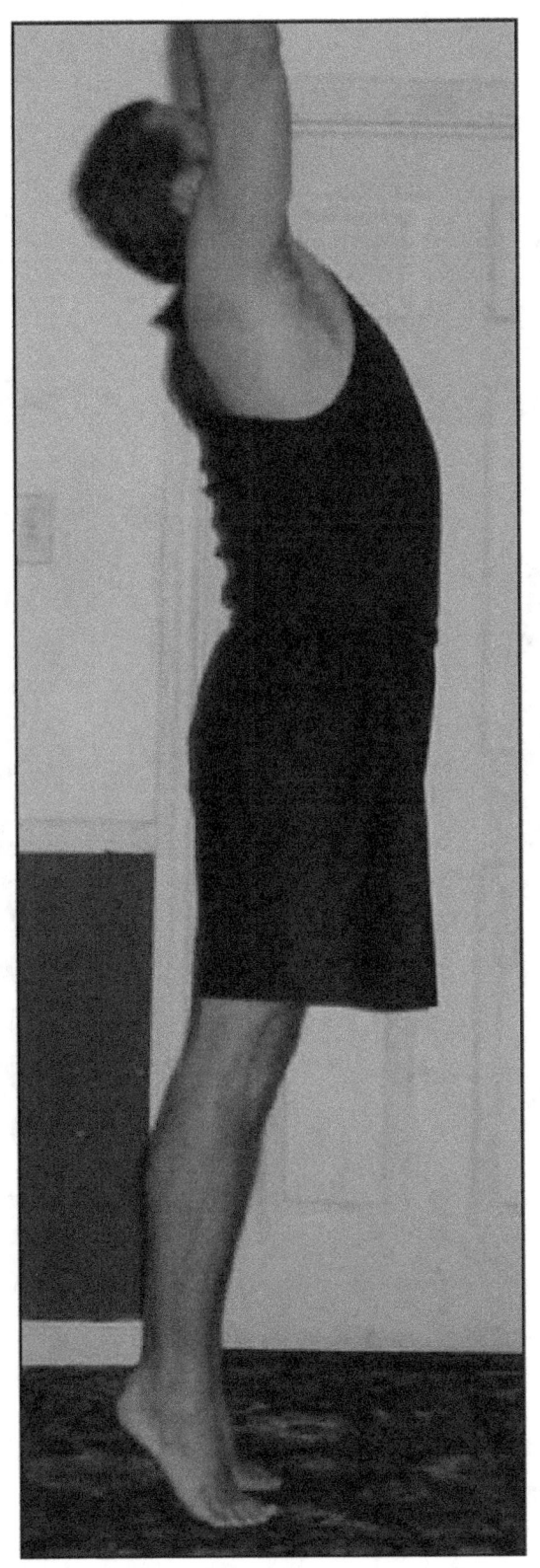

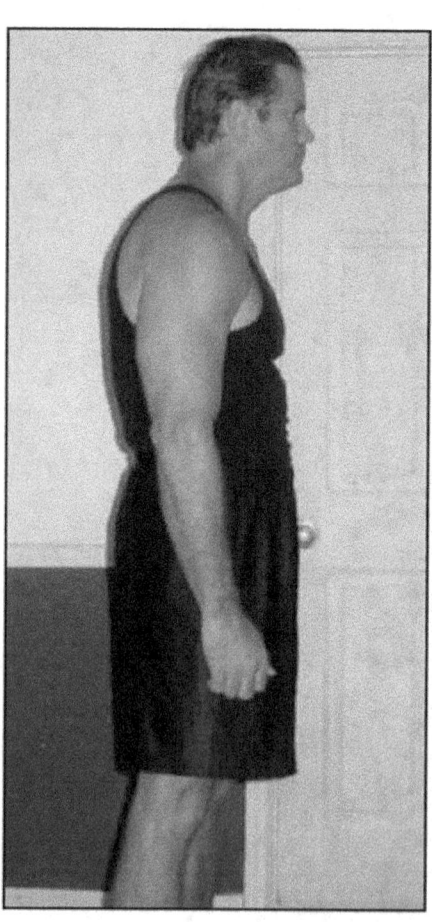

Stand tall and shrug the shoulders up and around to loosen them.

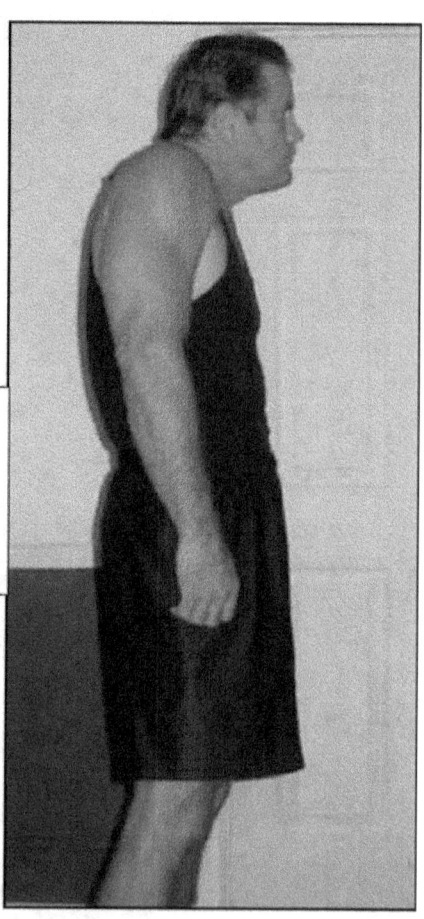

Ab Stretches

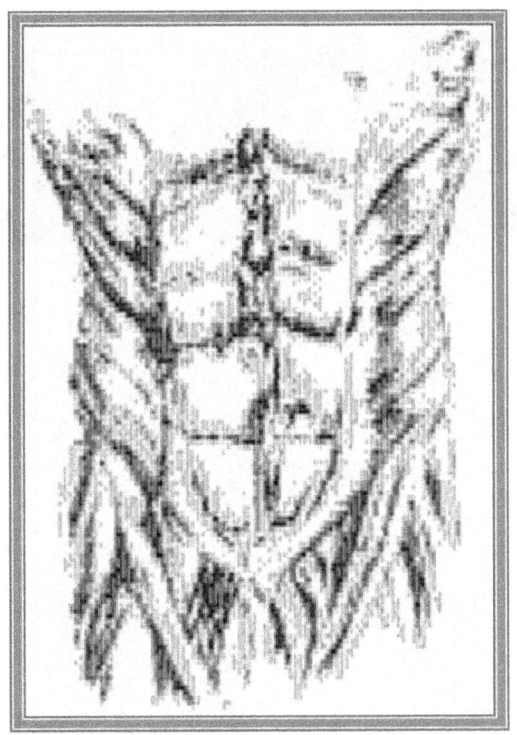

Do all stretches 6 to 8 times. Relax and breath easy, do not bounce or force the stretch..

The basic "crunch" Place the hands behind the head, feet on the ground and then lift the feet while pulling the body off the floor

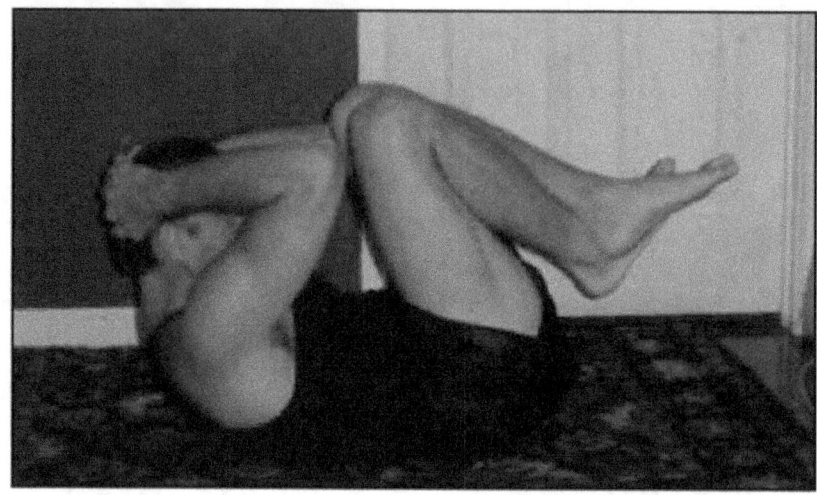

Reach up and grab the knees and pull the head towards the knee to stretch the back.

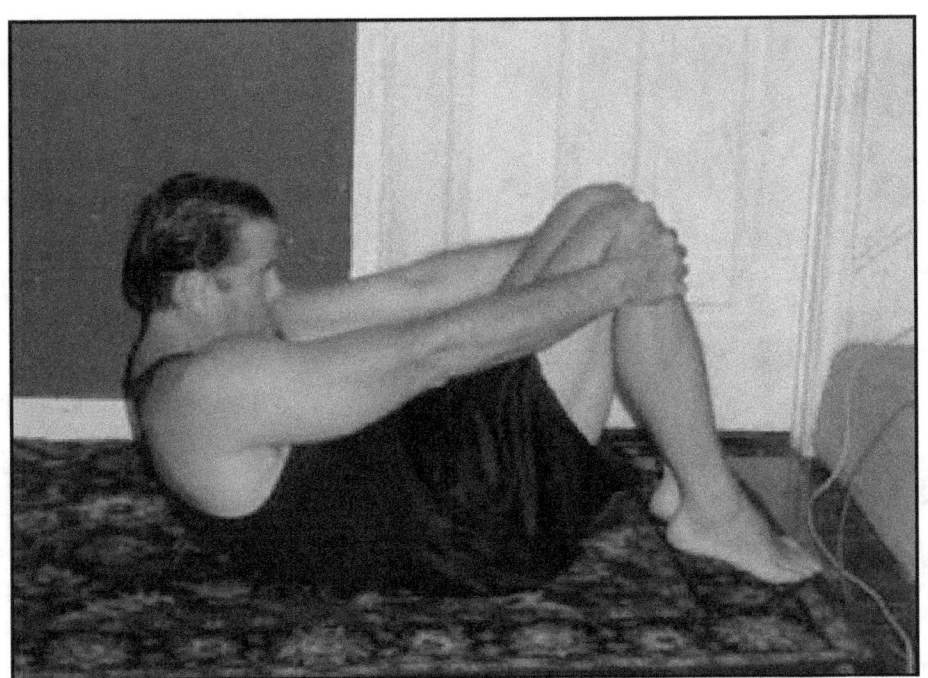

Modify the crunch by crossing the legs.

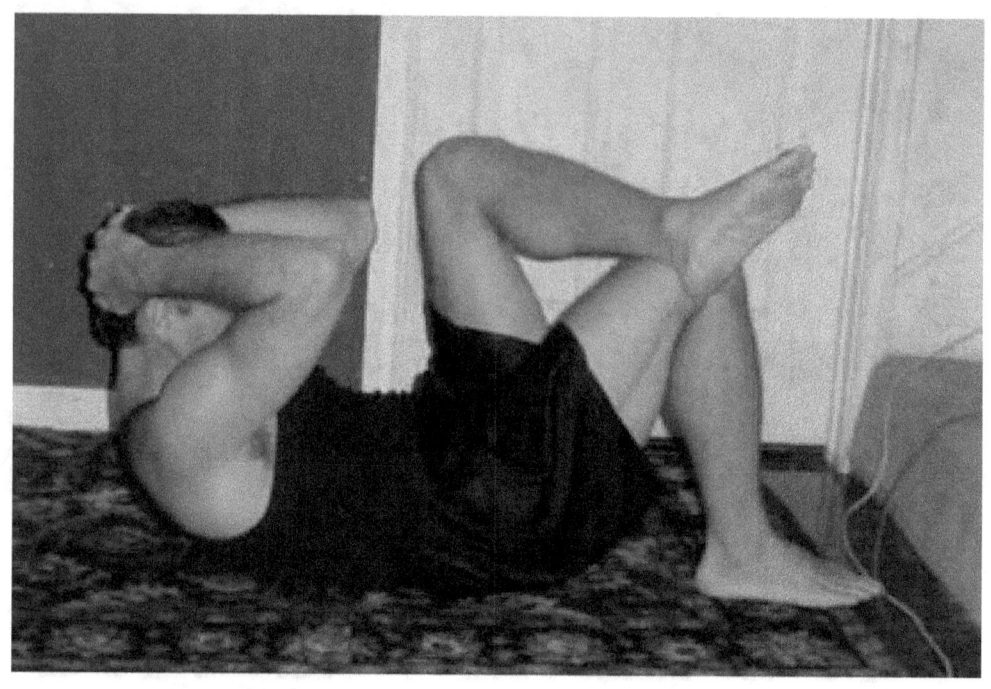

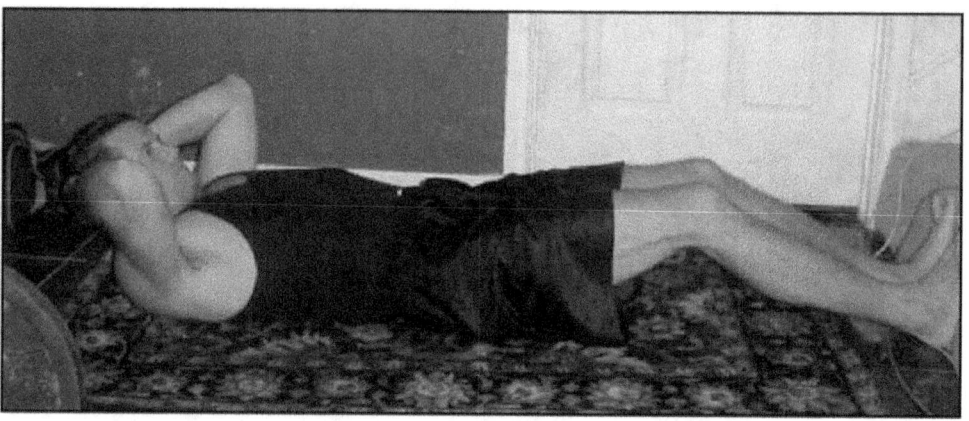

The basic stiff legged sit up with the hands behind the neck.

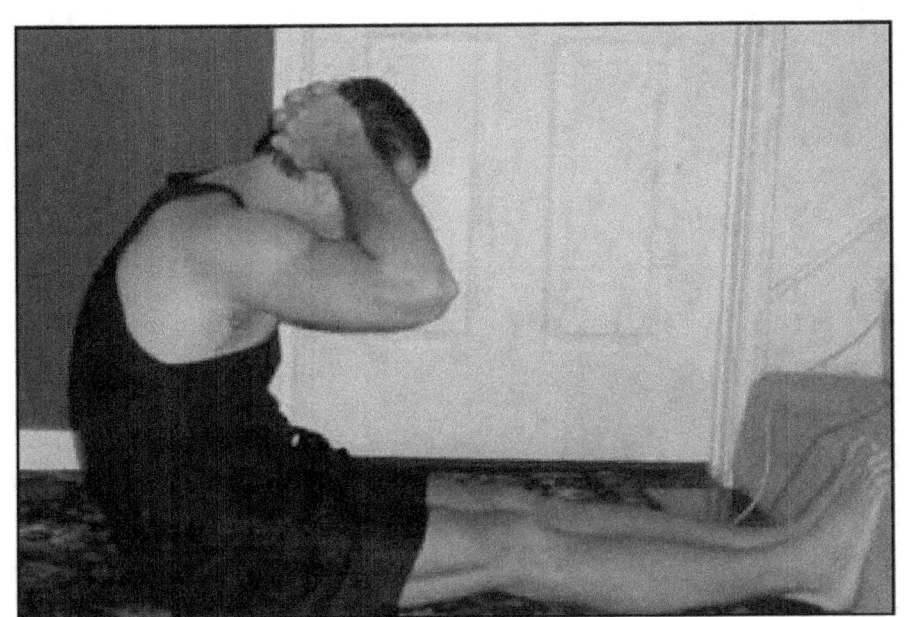

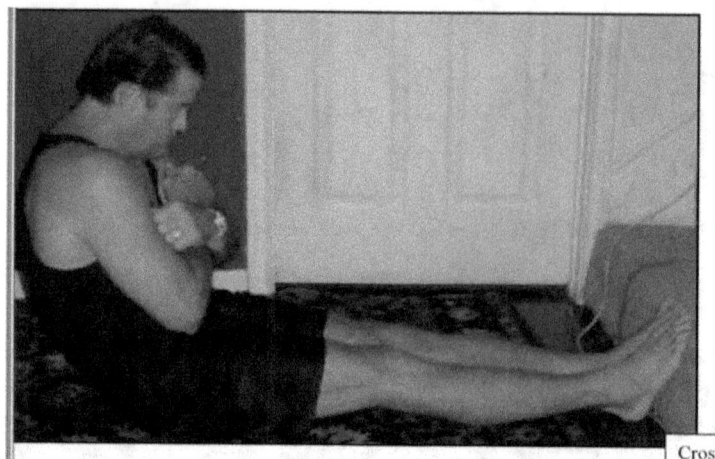

Cross the arms across the
body to modify the sit up.

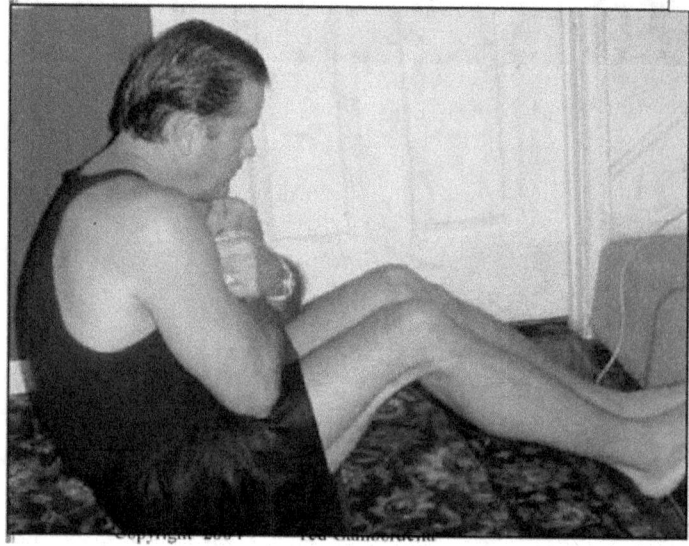

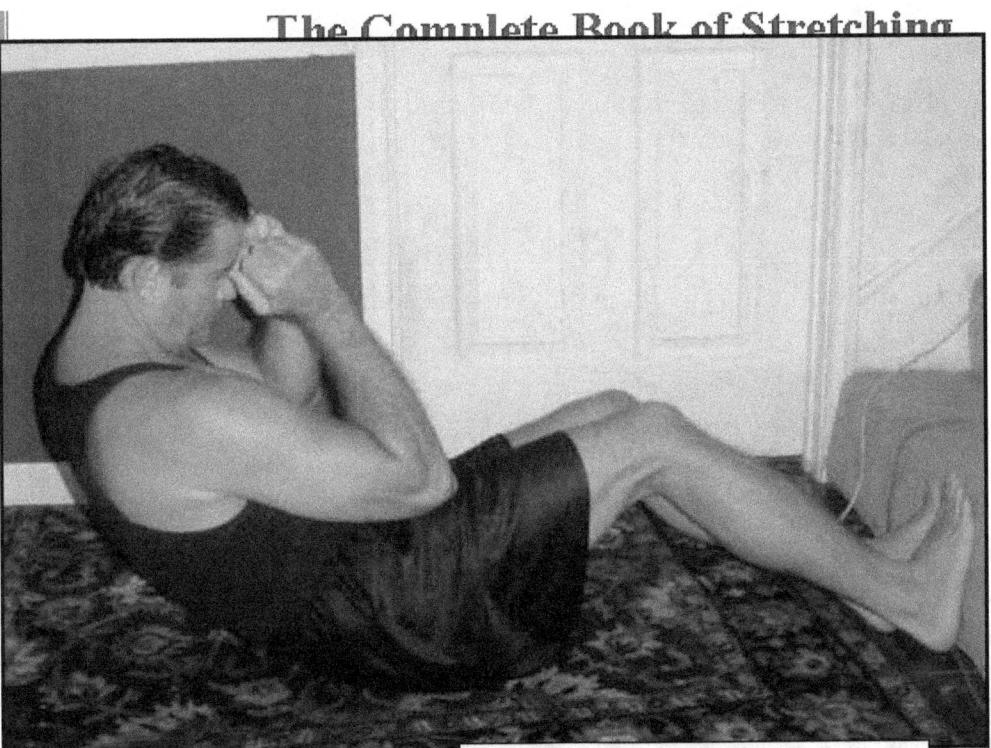

Here we work the side by doing a sit up and leaning to either side as we come up.

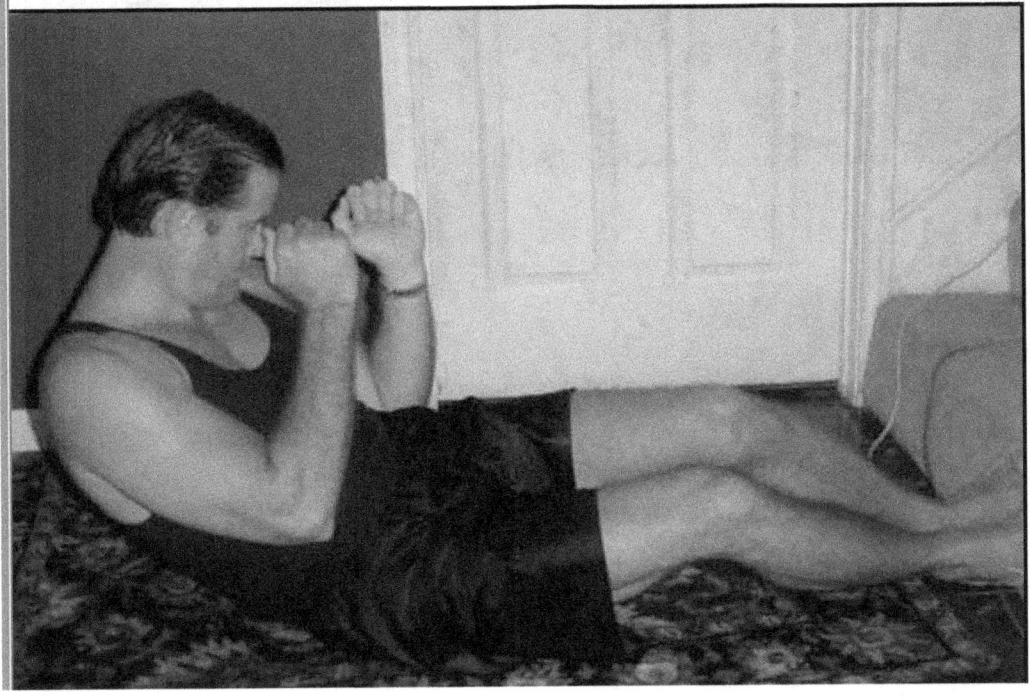

You can stretch the hips by lying on your side and lifting the leg straight up.

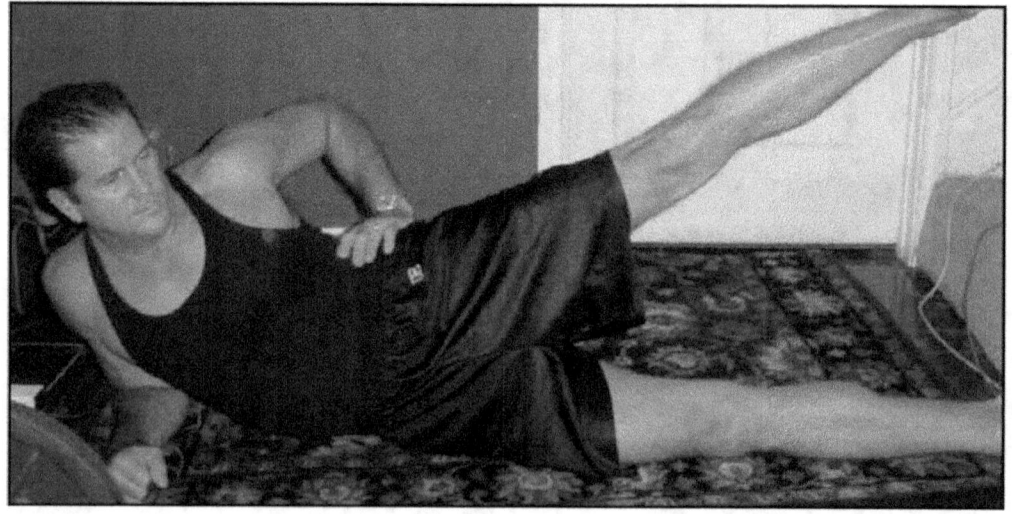

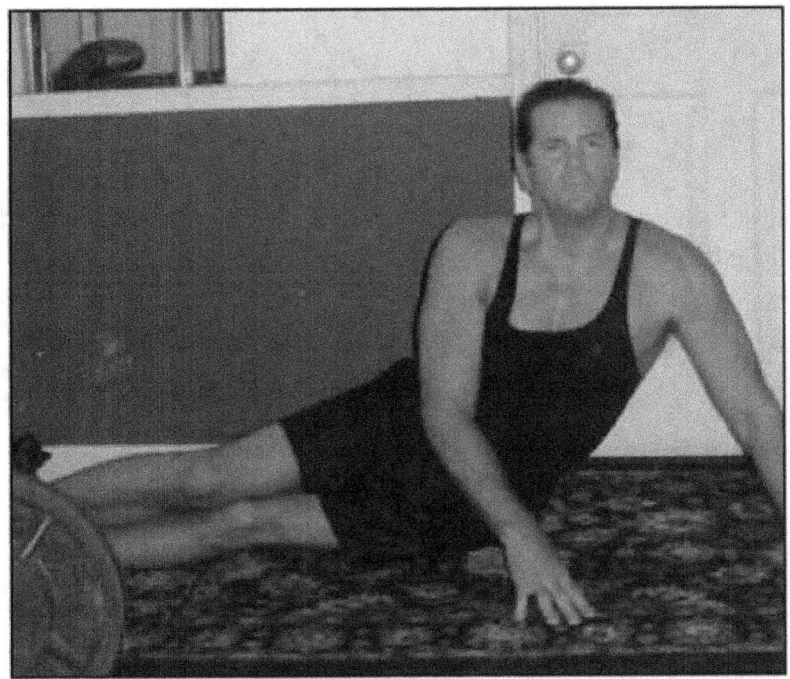

Lie on the floor on your side and then supported by your hands arch the body up to the side.

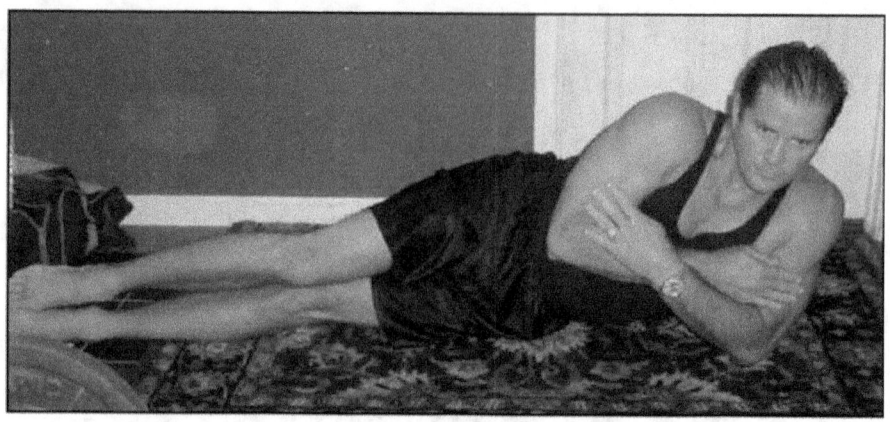

You can also arch the body up to the side with using only the side muscles by crossing the arms.

Arm Stretches

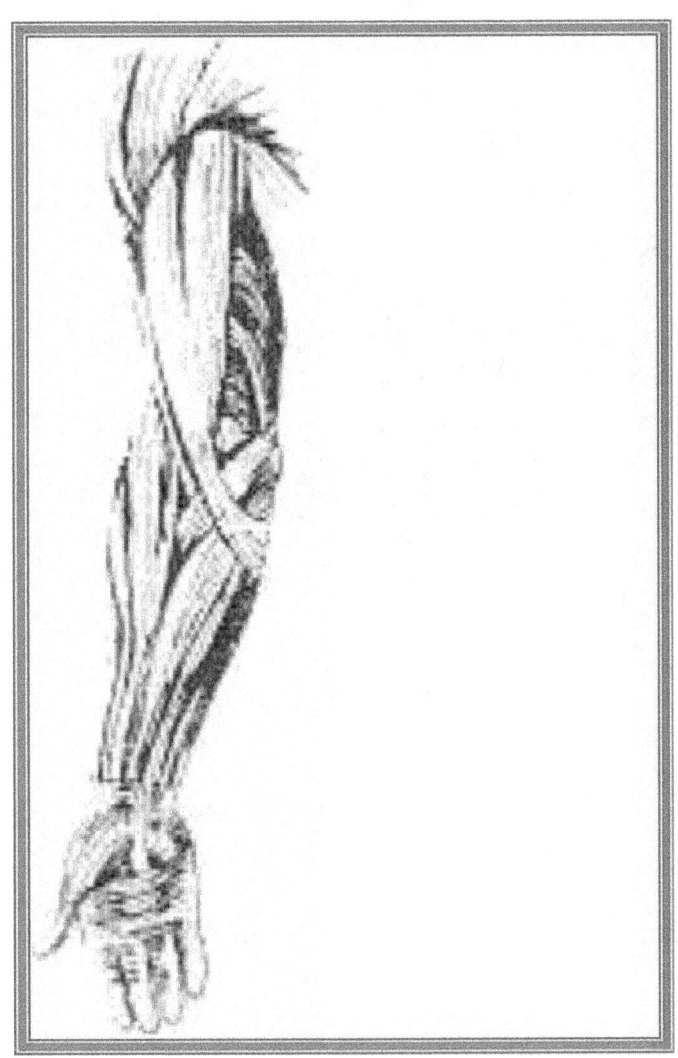

Do all stretches 6 to 8 times. Relax and breath easy, do not bounce or force the stretch..

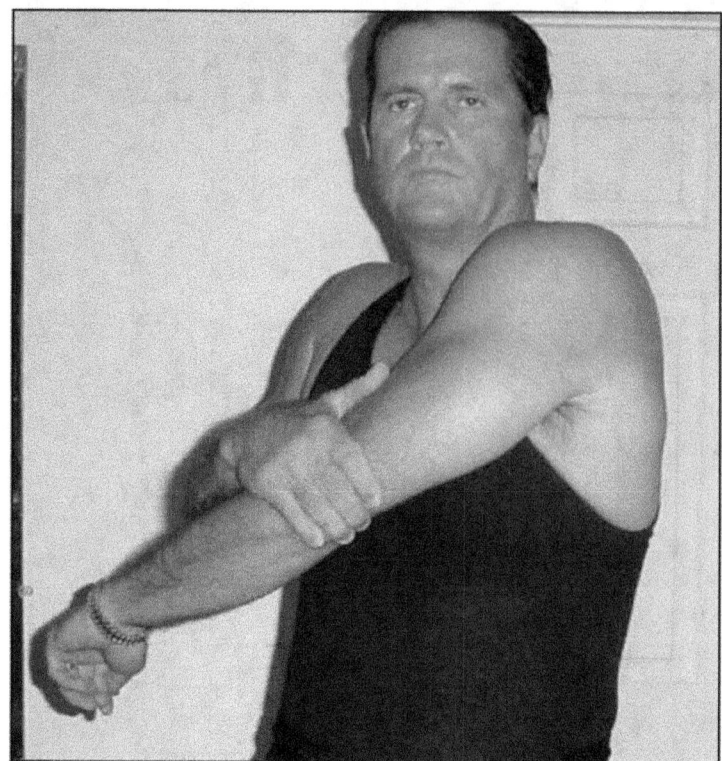

Reach across the body and grab the elbow. Pull it gently across your body.

reach behind your body and grab the wrist of one arm, gently pull the wrist behind your back.

While holding your wrist with the other arm lean forward to stretch. Repeat to both sides.

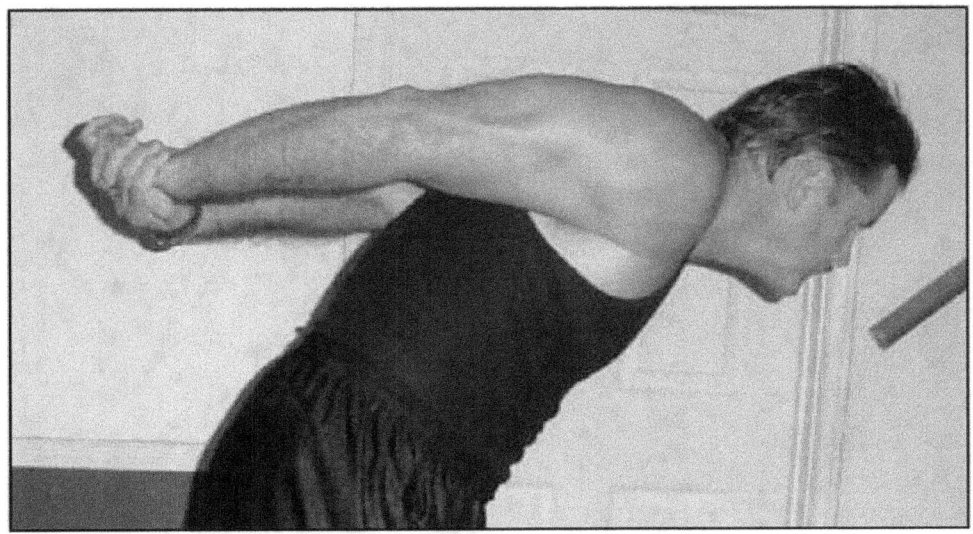

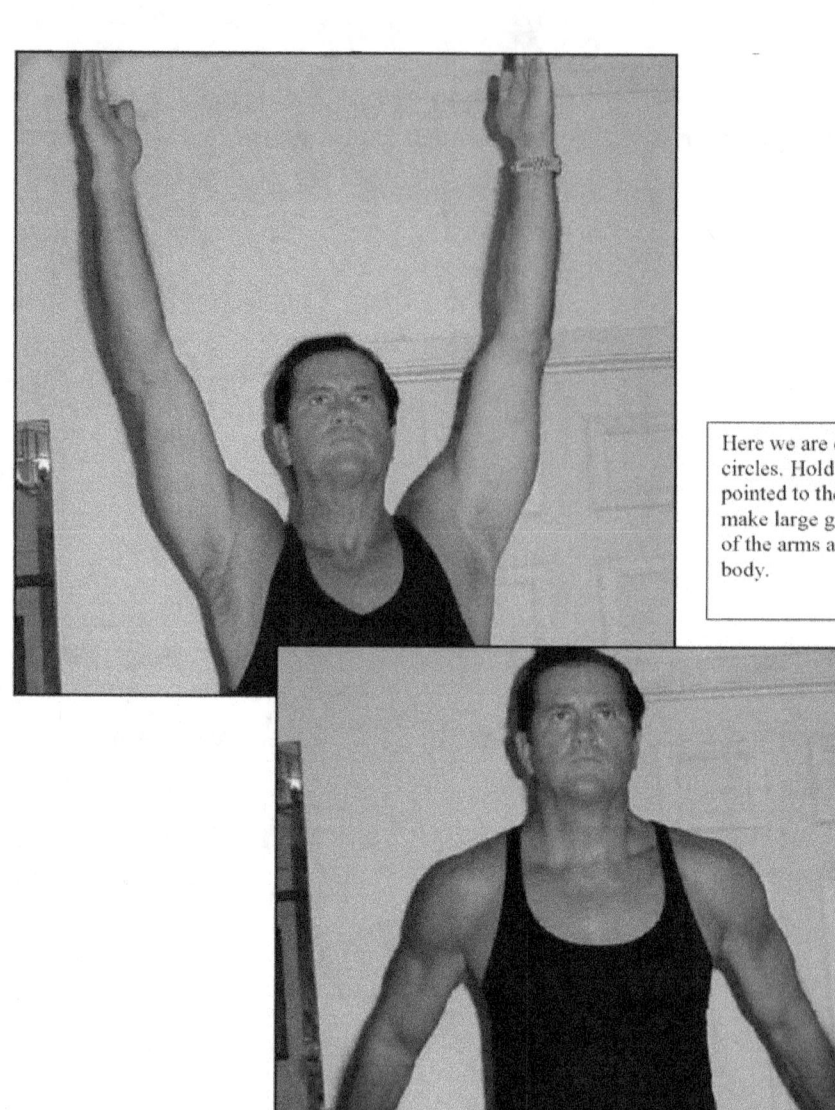

Here we are doing arm circles. Hold the hands pointed to the sides and make large gentle swings of the arms around the body.

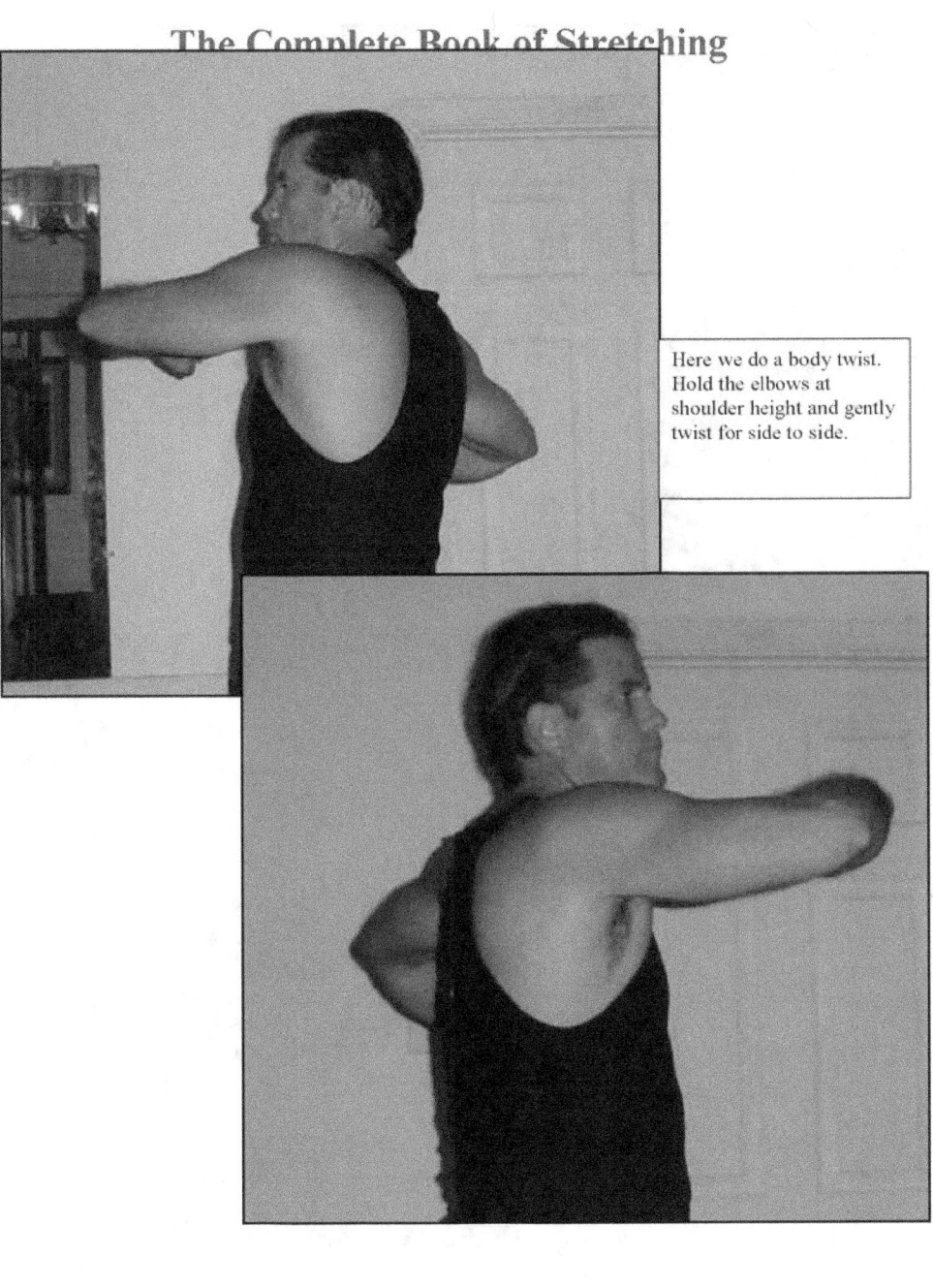

Here we do a body twist. Hold the elbows at shoulder height and gently twist for side to side.

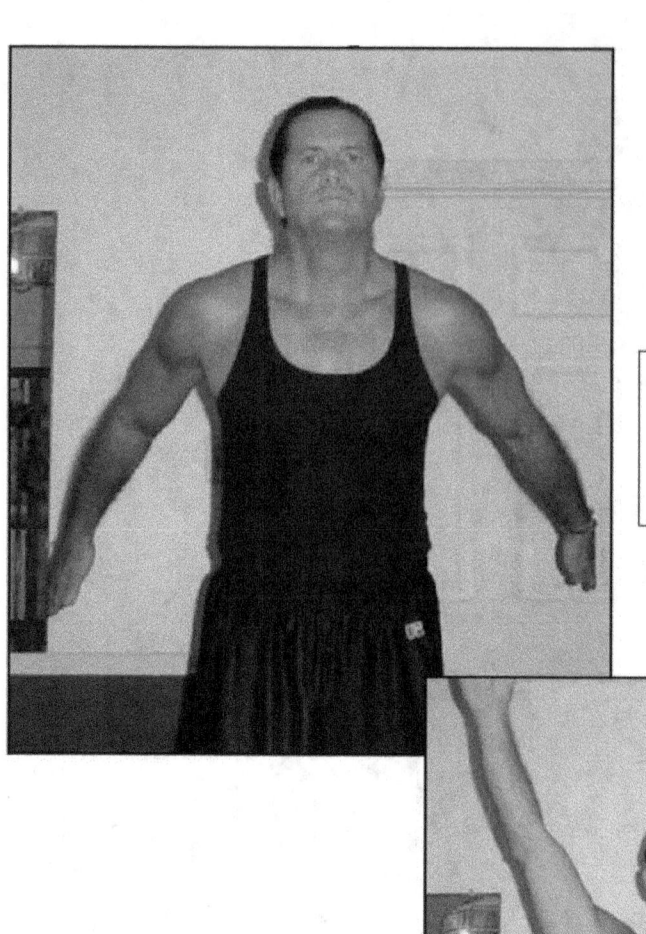

Here we do a modified arm swing. Hold the arms straight to the sides and swing them up as high as possible to the front.

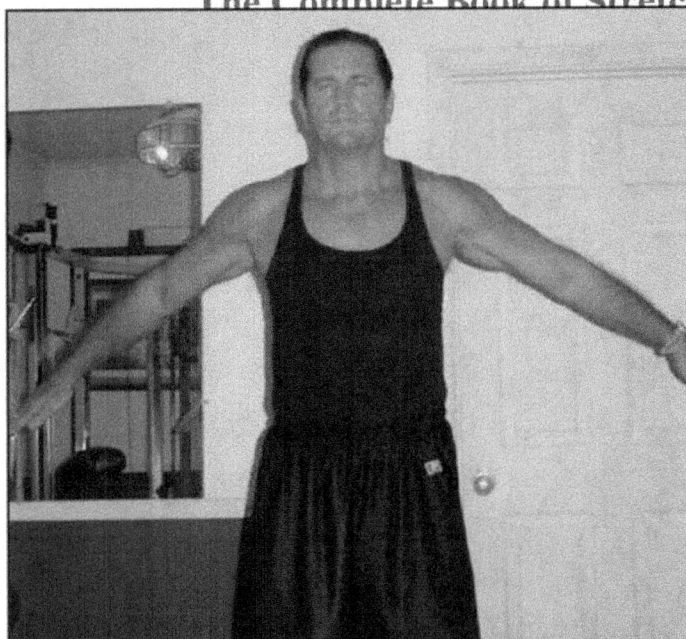

Small arm circles, holding the arms to the side make small circles forward and backwards..

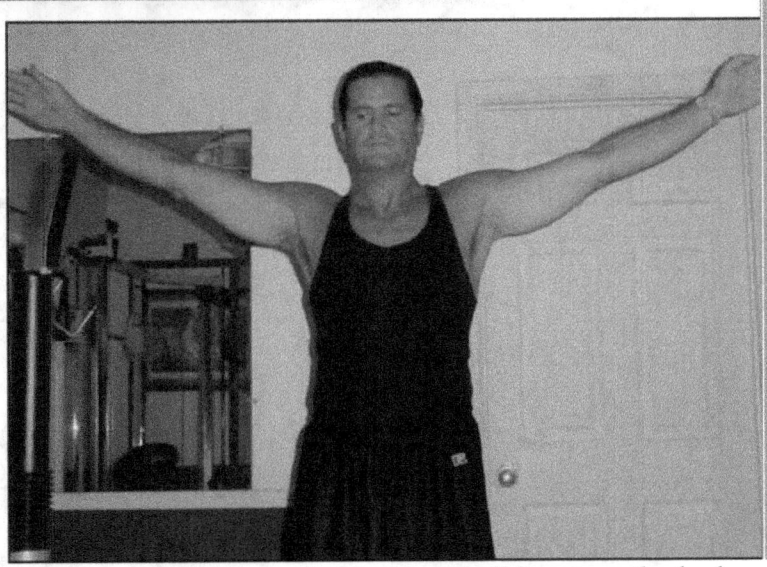

Reach up and grab the tricep of the opposite arm and pull it across the body.

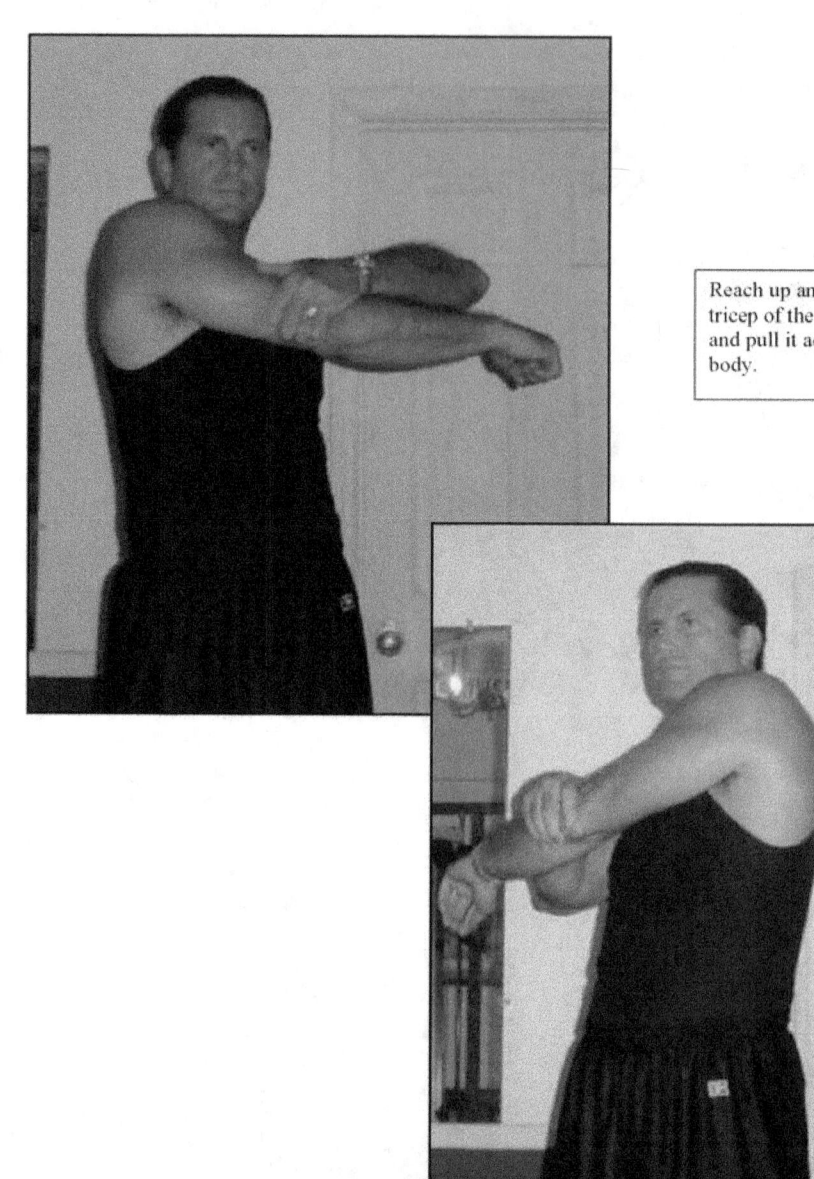

Reach up and grab t
tricep of the opposit
and pull it across th
body.

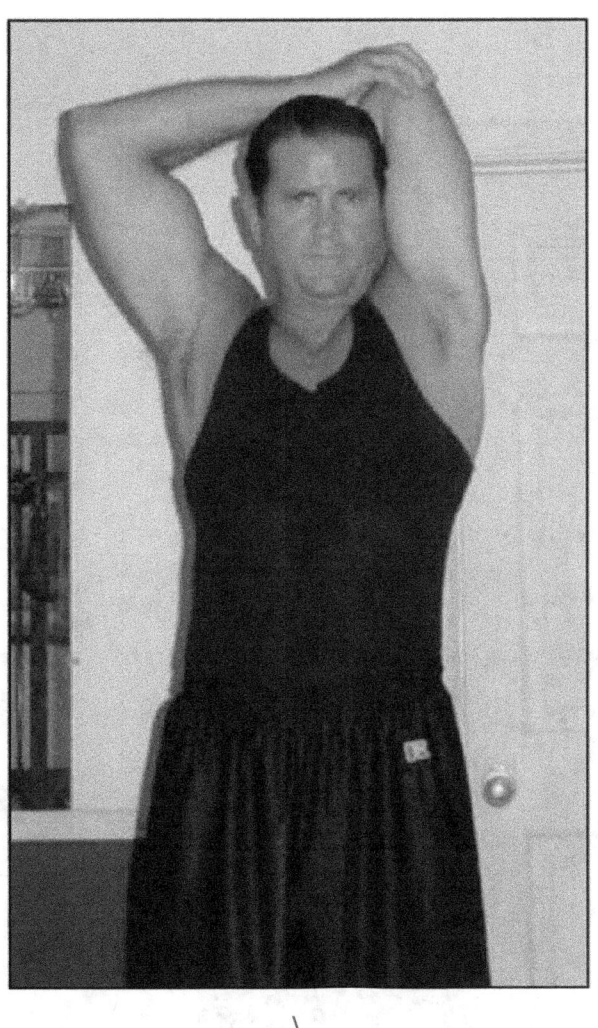

Reach up and grab the tricep of the opposite arm and pull it across the body.

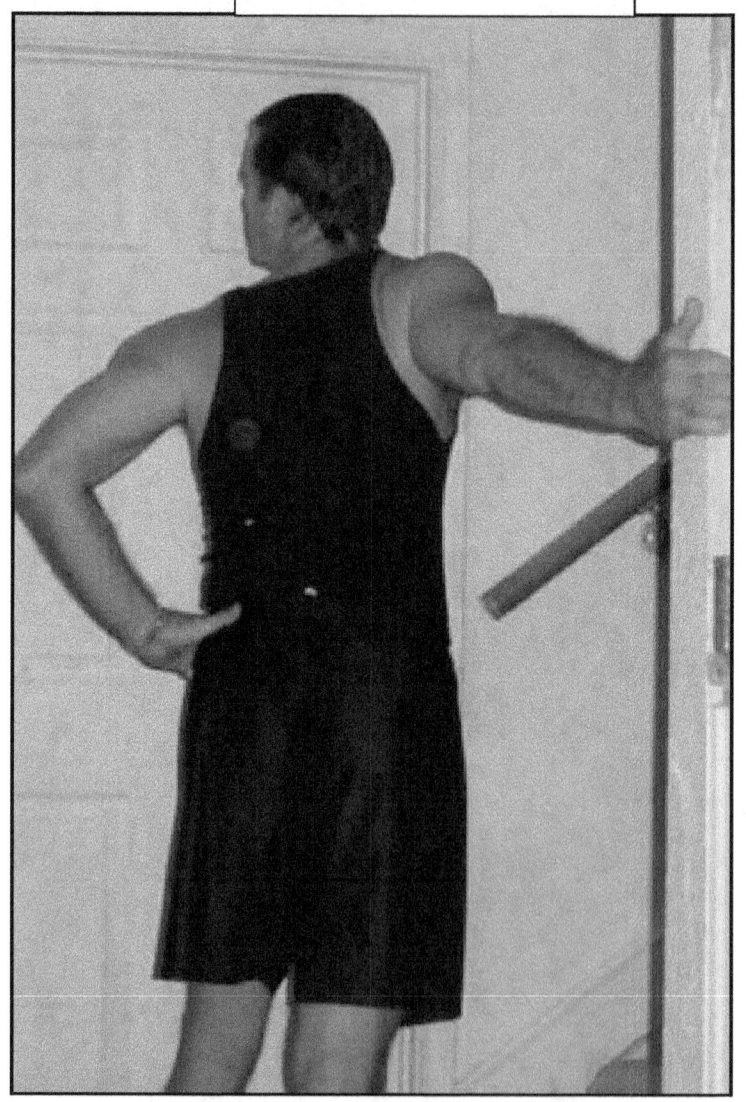

Reach out and hold the wall while pulling the body forward.

Here we stretch wrist and fingers by placing the hand flat on the bench and pushing down with the palm of the other hand..

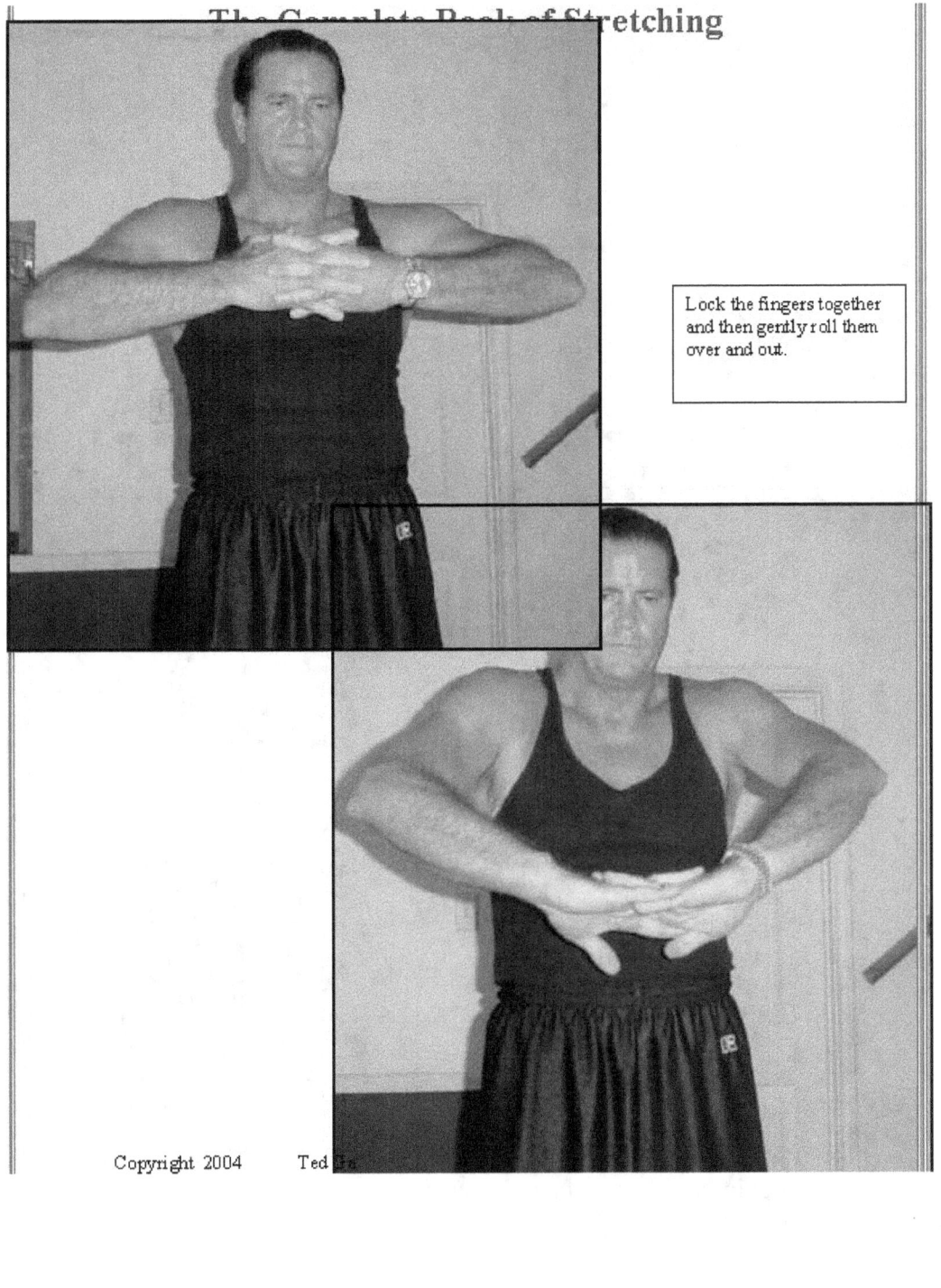

Lock the fingers together
and then gently roll them
over and out.

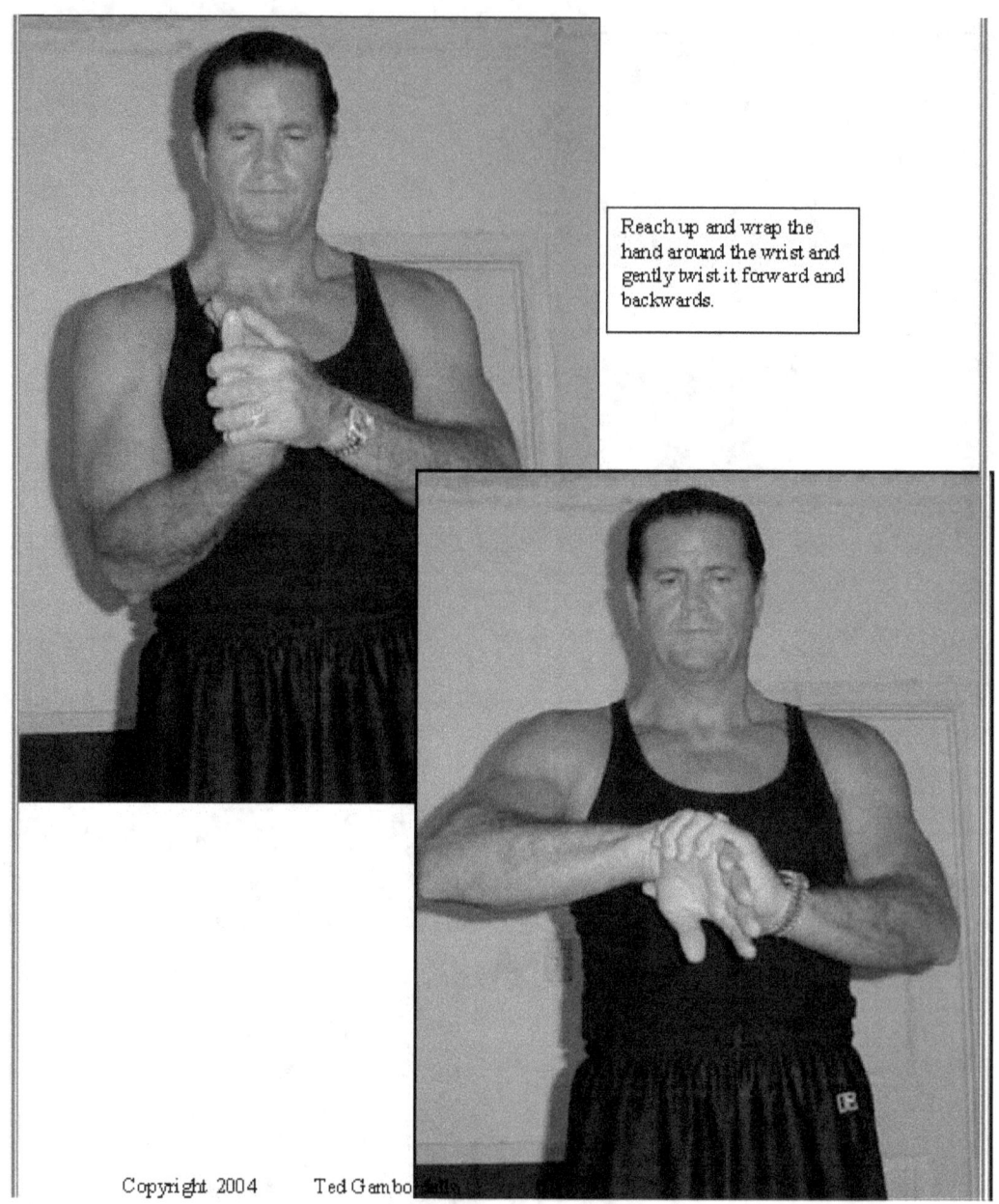

Reach up and wrap the hand around the wrist and gently twist it forward and backwards.

Hold the wrist pointed down and gently push on the back of the wrist with the other hand. Hold the hands together as if praying in front of the head and then drop them down in front of the body.

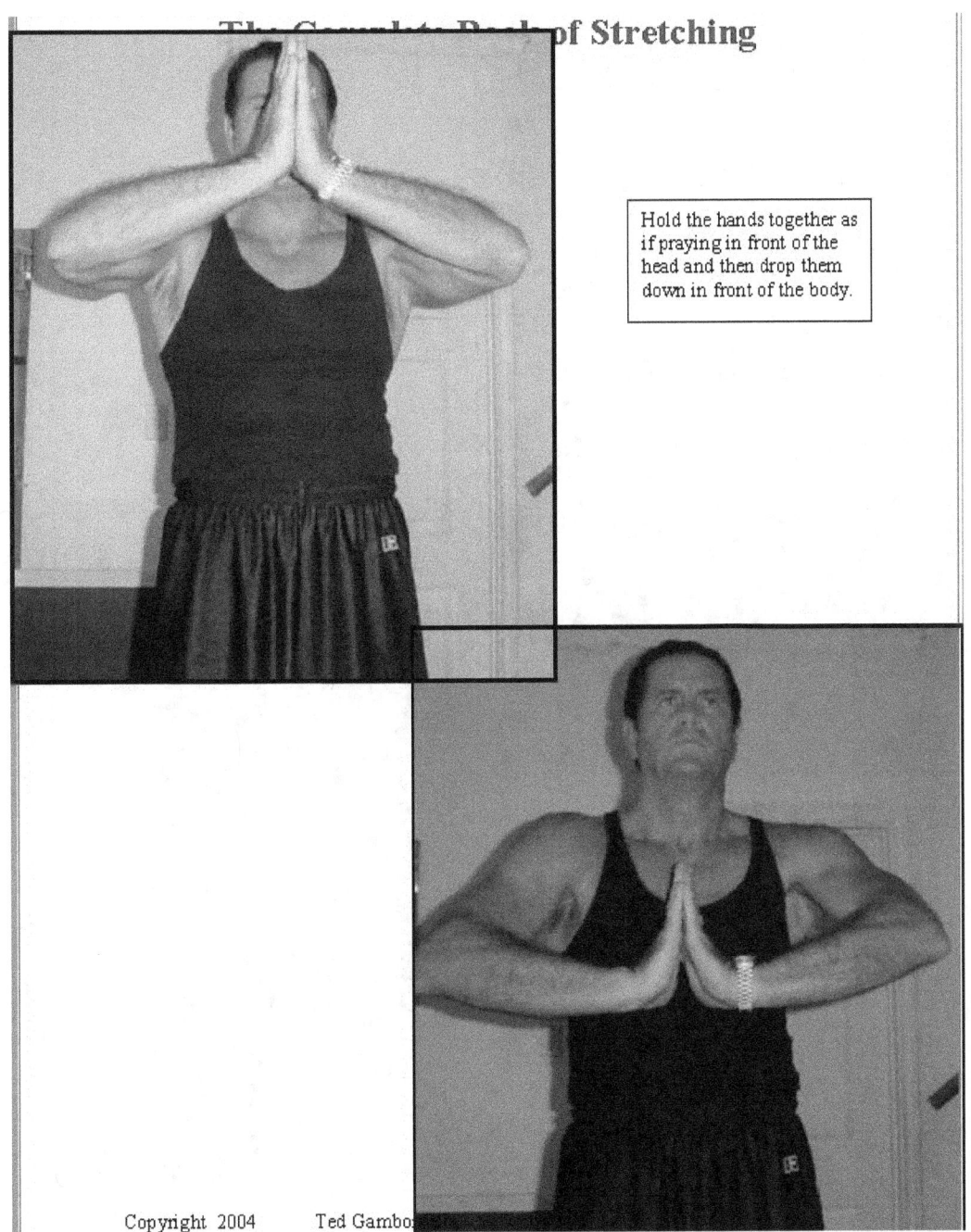

Hold the hands together as if praying in front of the head and then drop them down in front of the body.

This is hard wrist twist, lock the fingers together and then roll the hand in a circle until the wrists are pointing forward.

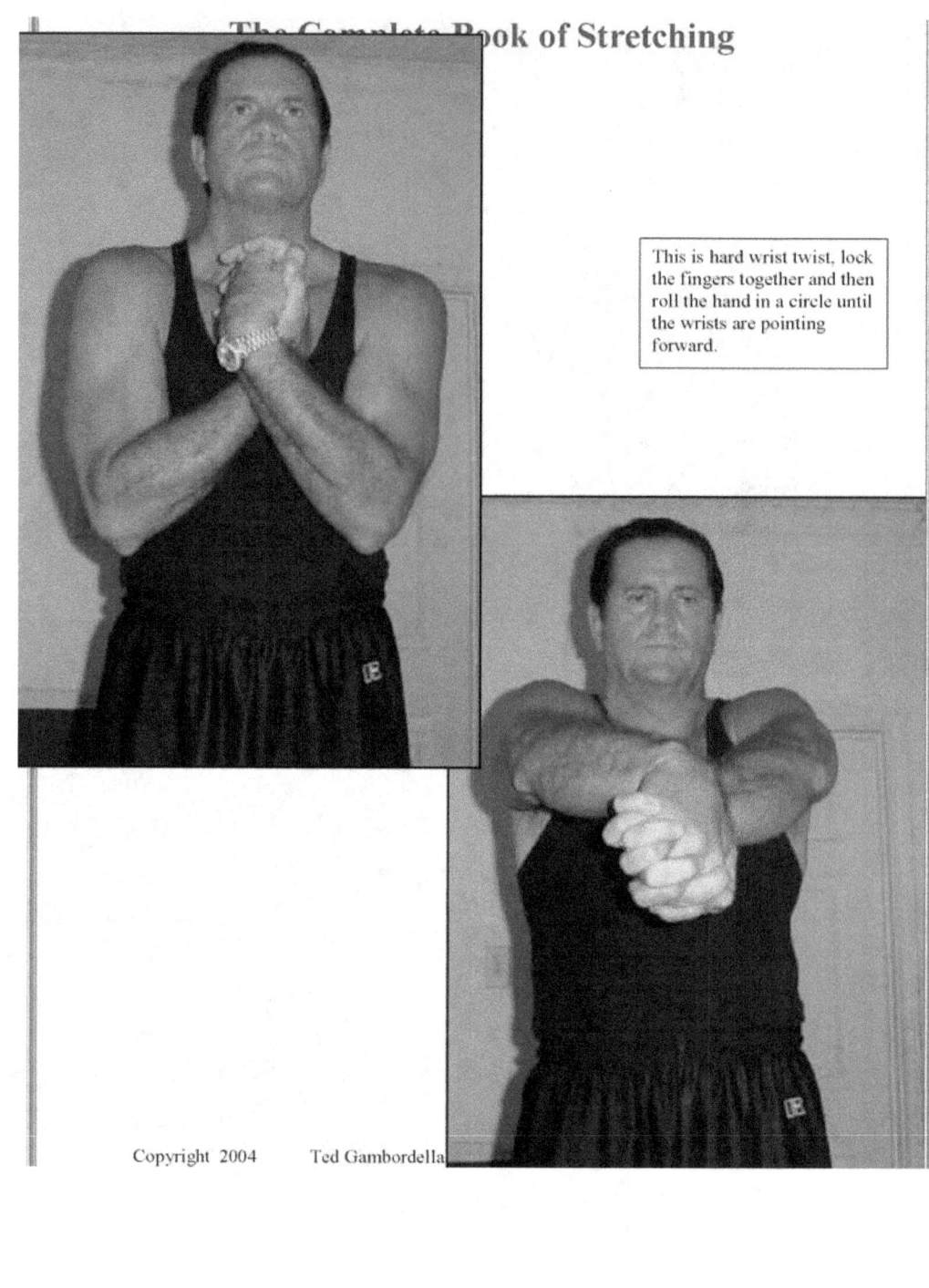

This is hard wrist twist, lock the fingers together and then roll the hand in a circle until the wrists are pointing forward.

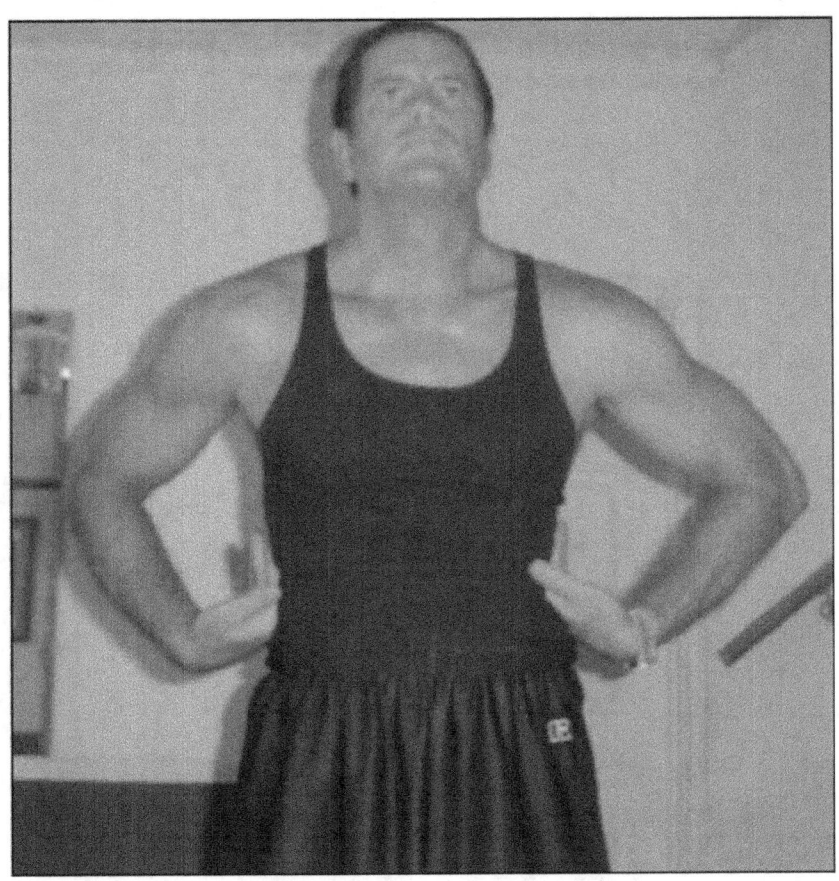

Here we stretch the wrists by placing them on the hips and pushing them gently into the body.

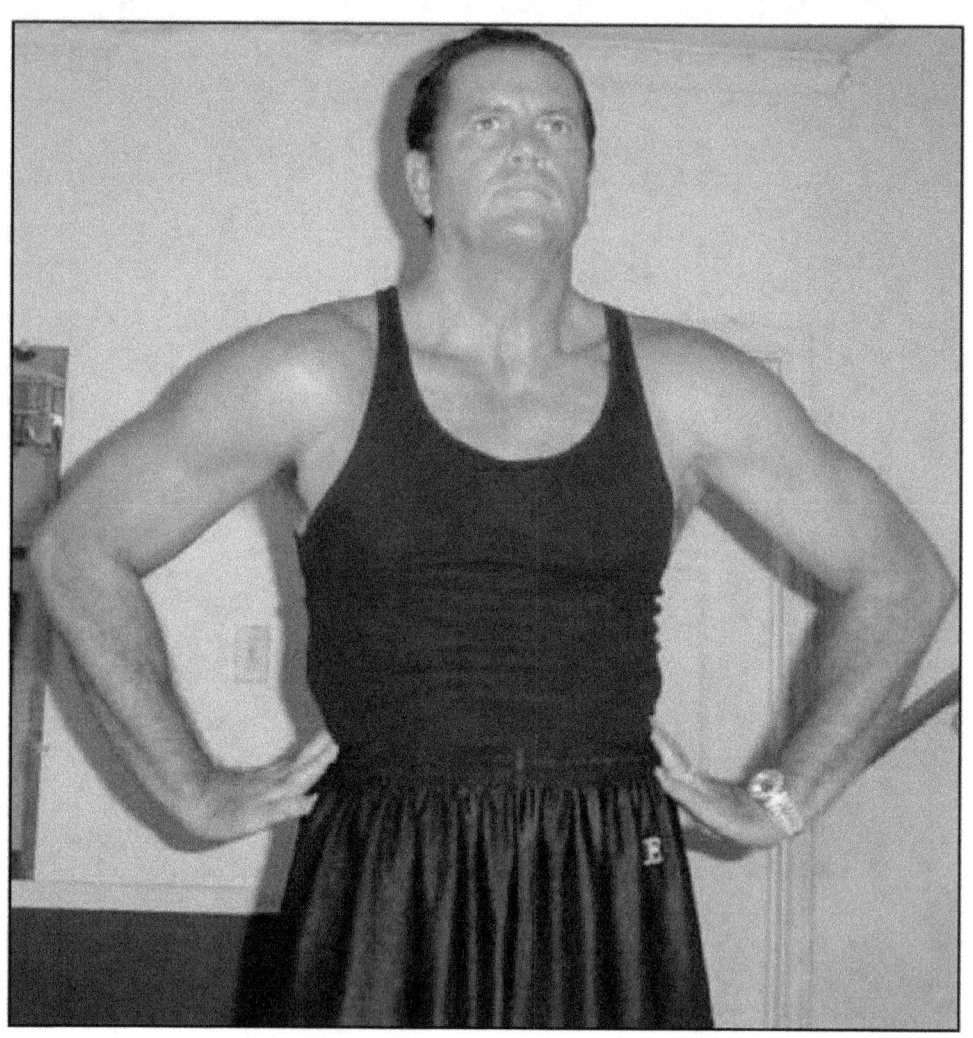

The same wrist stretch done with the palms facing down.

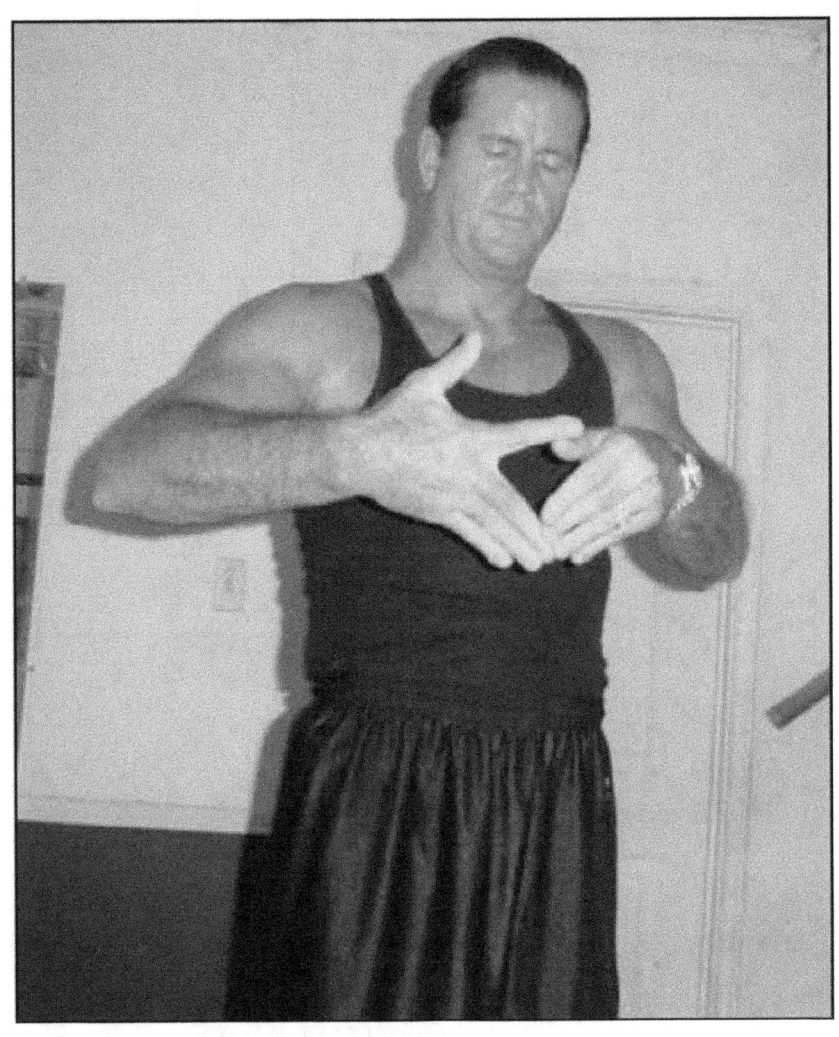

Here we stretch the fingers by gently pulling them apart.
Another finger stretch, were we reach down and grab the fingers and gently bend
them backwards. We can also do all 4 fingers at once.

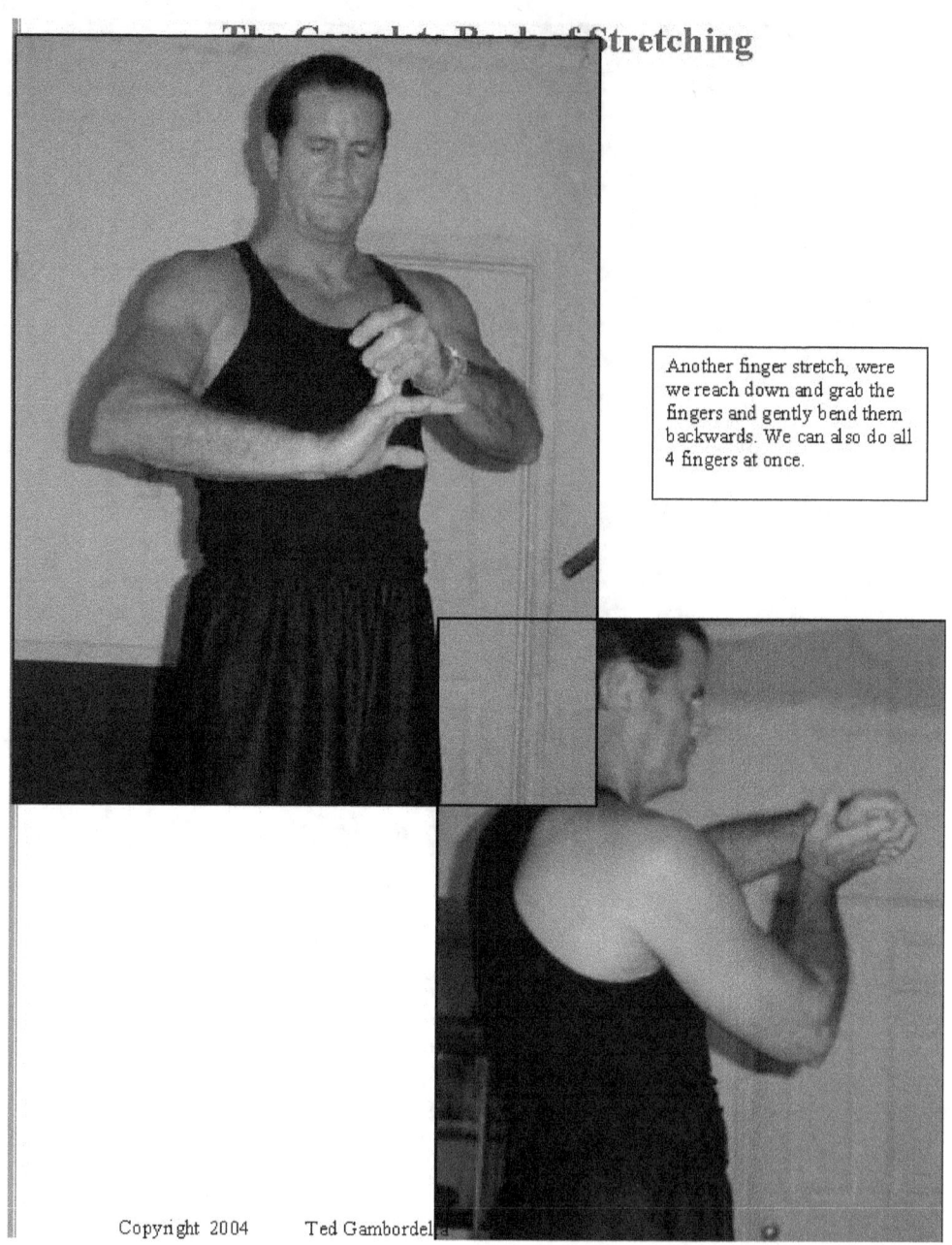

Another finger stretch, were we reach down and grab the fingers and gently bend them backwards. We can also do all 4 fingers at once.

Here we stretch the wrist by grabbing it and turning it over.

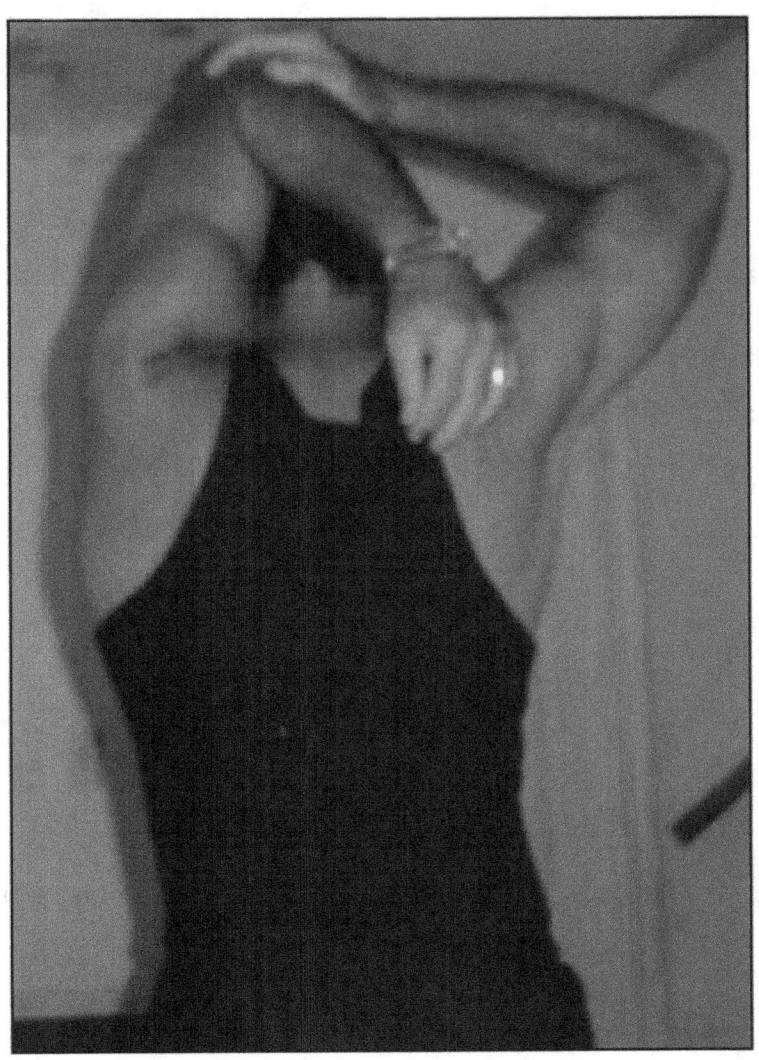

Reach up and grab the tricep of the opposite arm and pull it down across the back.

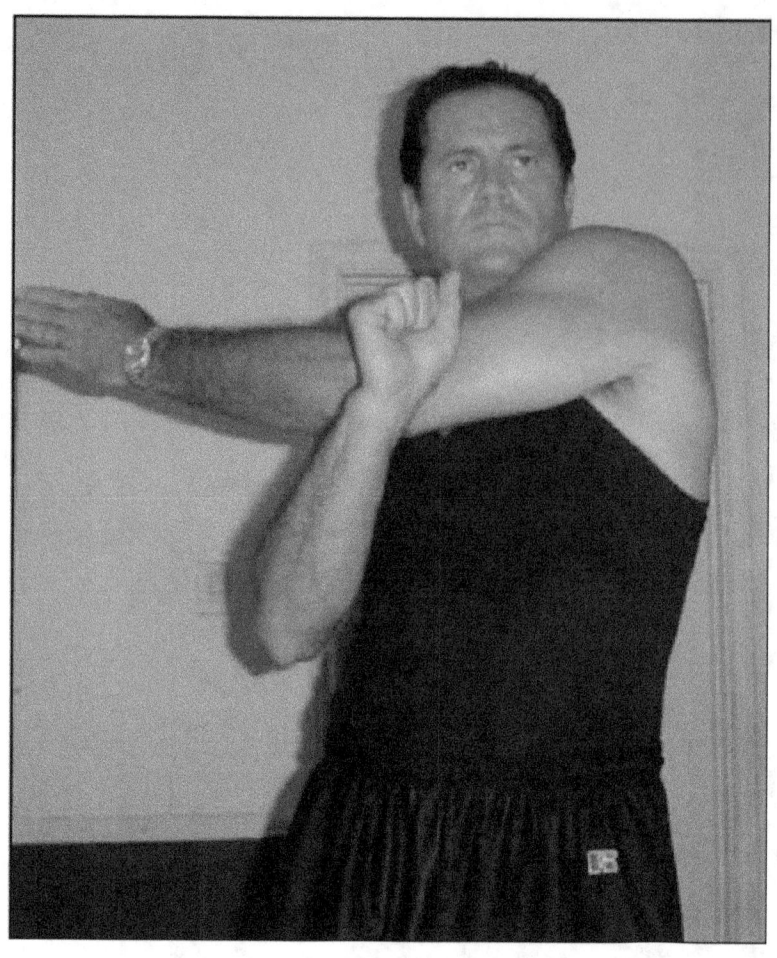

Reach up and grab the tricep of the opposite arm and pull it across the body.

Reach around and grab the wrist of one arm with the other, then lean forward and stretch it.

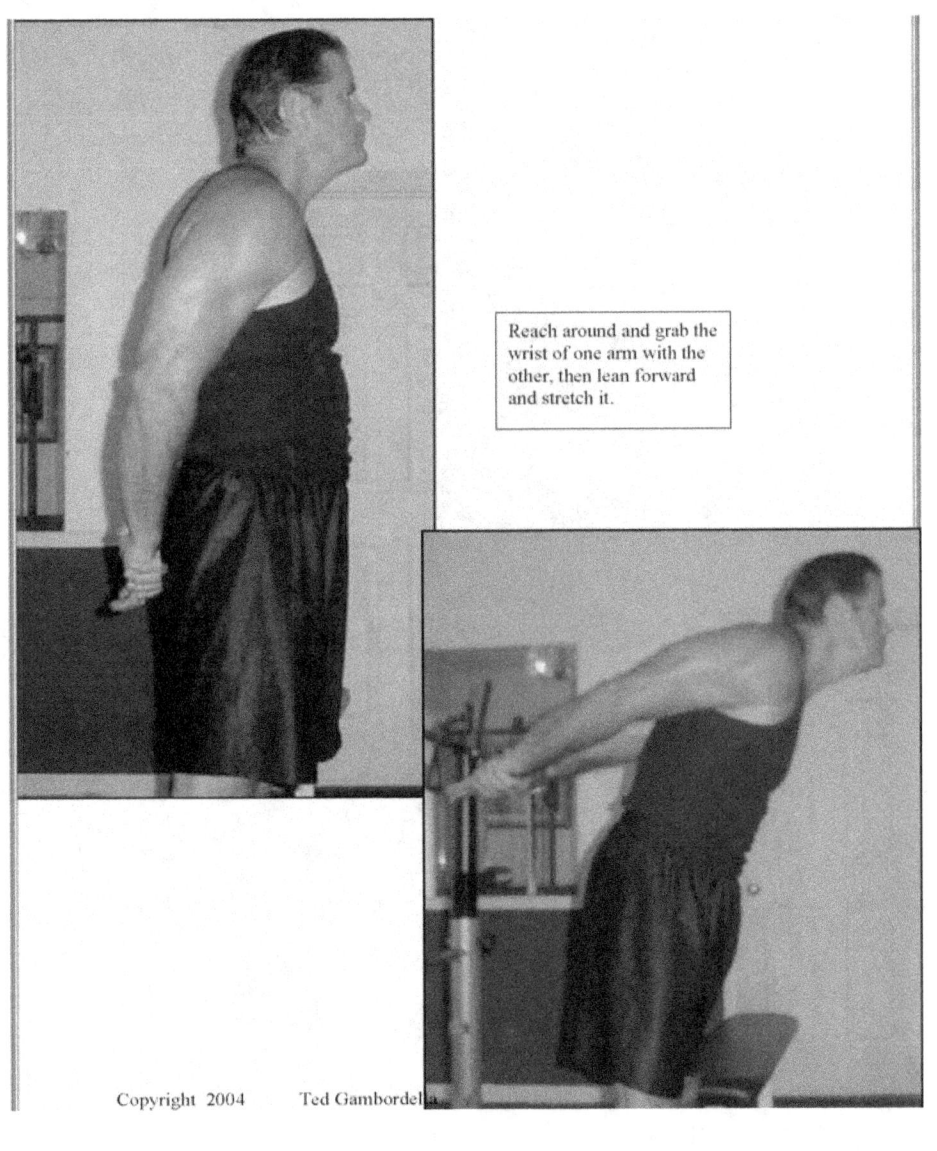

Reach around and grab the wrist of one arm with the other, then lean forward and stretch it.

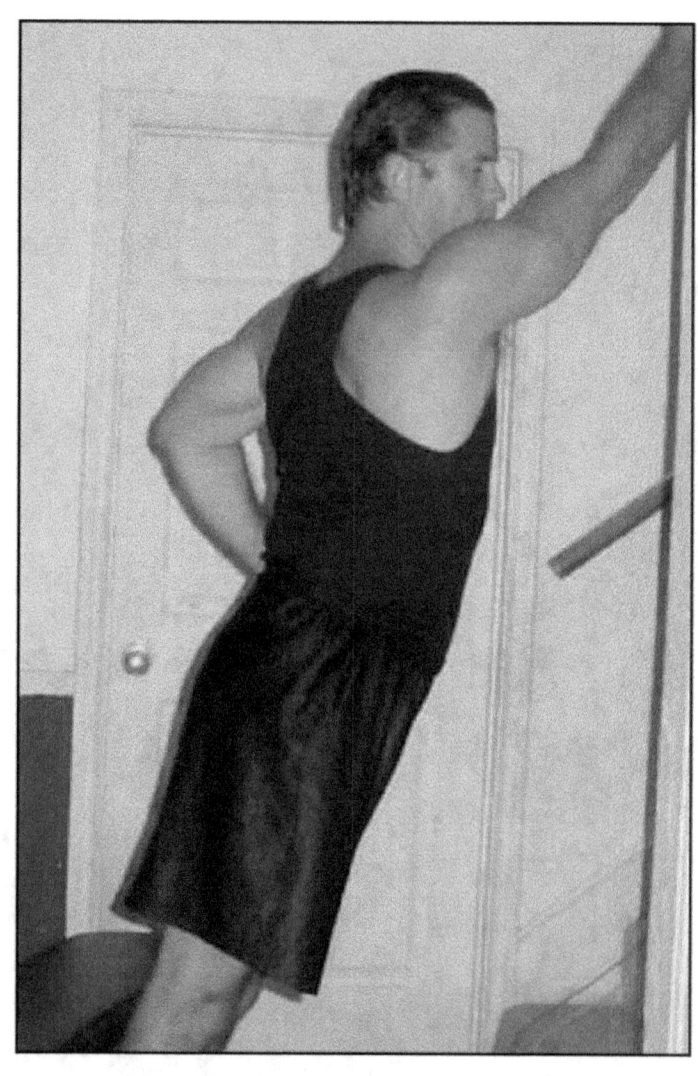

Lean out to the wall and hold one arm on the wall and you stretch forward.

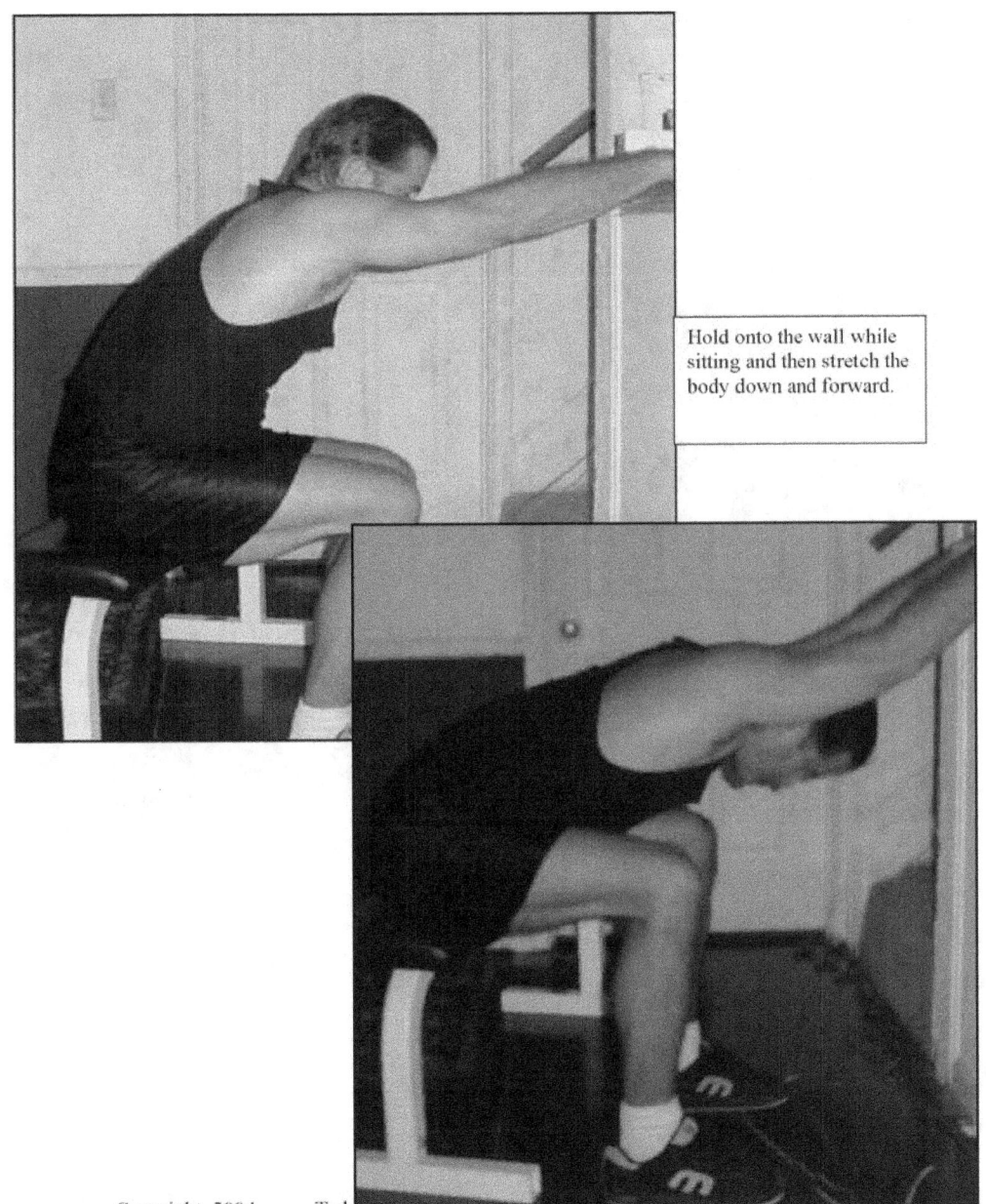

Hold onto the wall while sitting and then stretch the body down and forward.

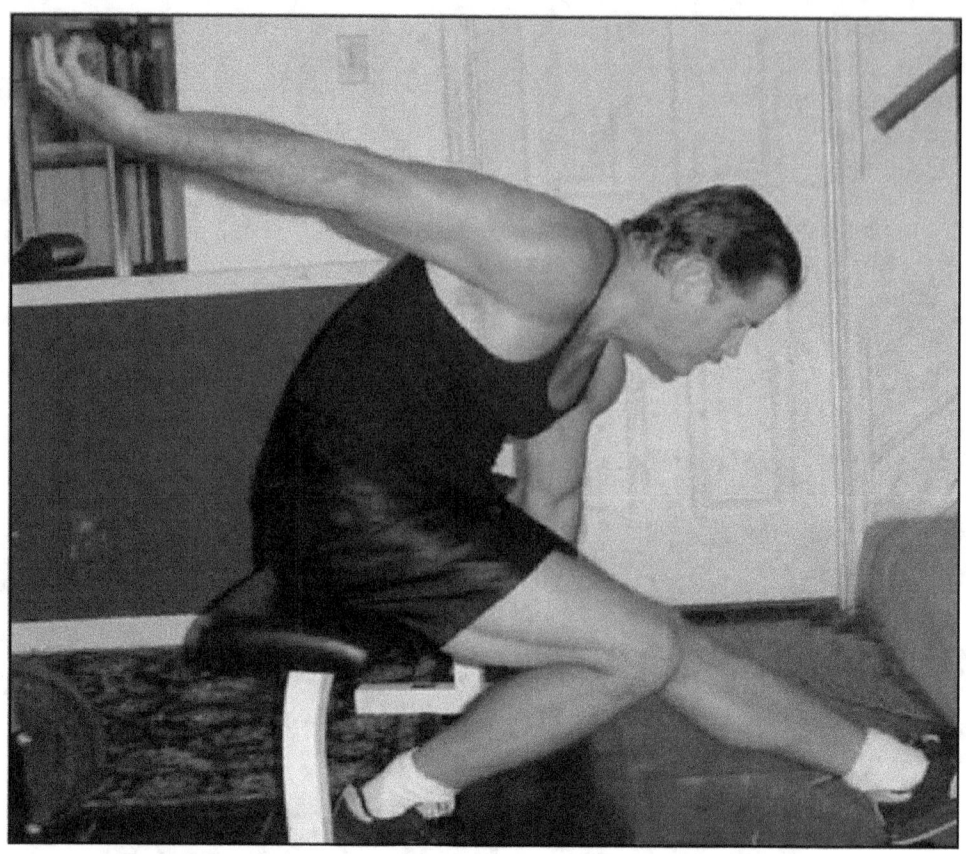

Put one leg straight out while sitting and reach back with the opposite arm. Alternate arms.

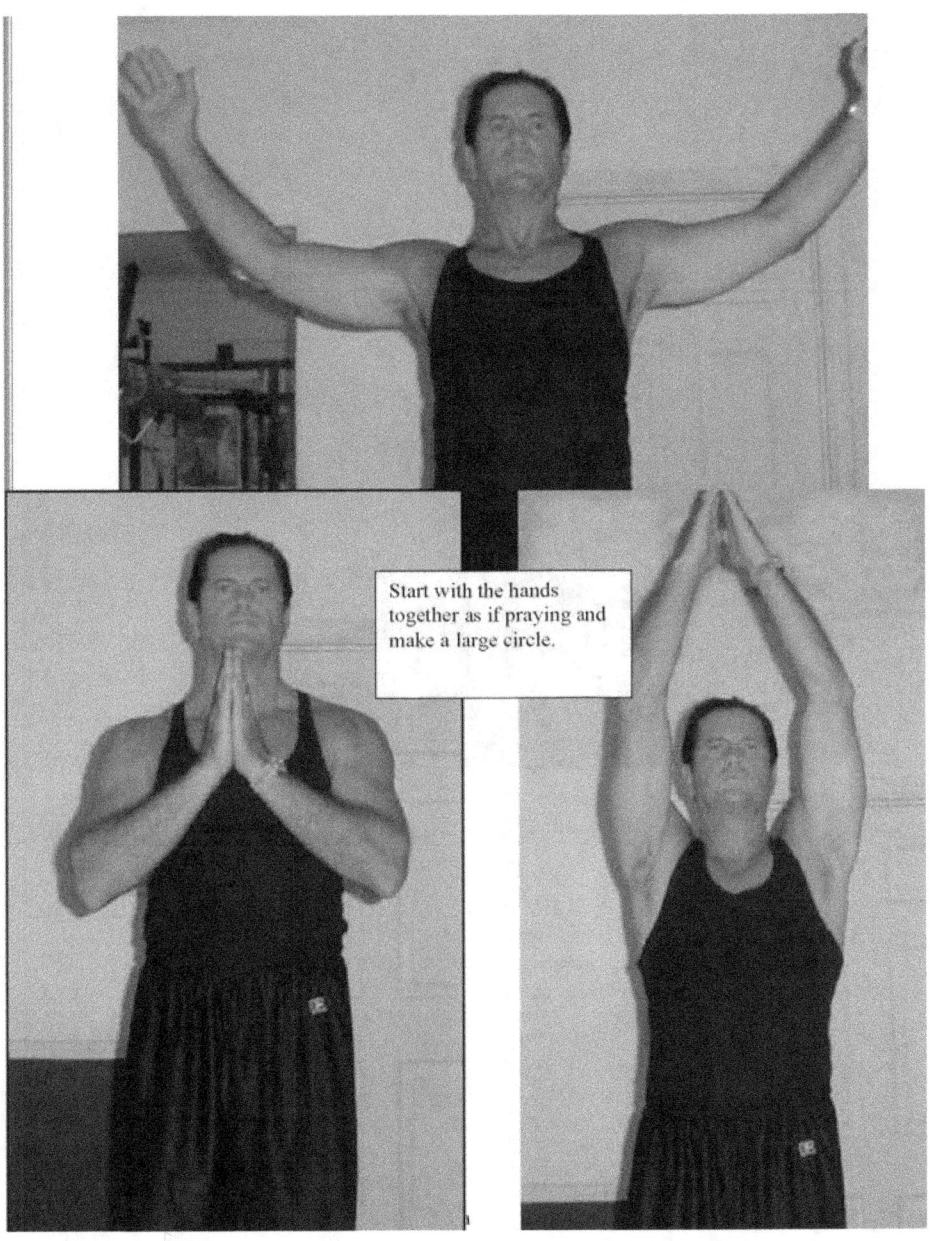

Start with the hands together as if praying and make a large circle.

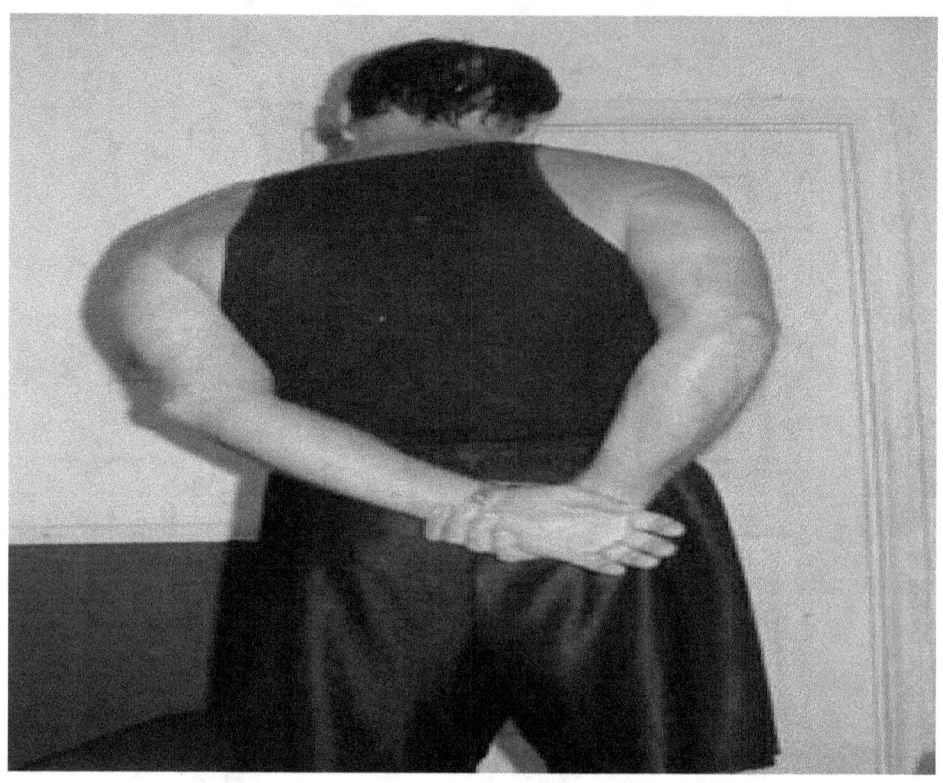

Reach back and grab the wrist and pull the arm across the back of the body.

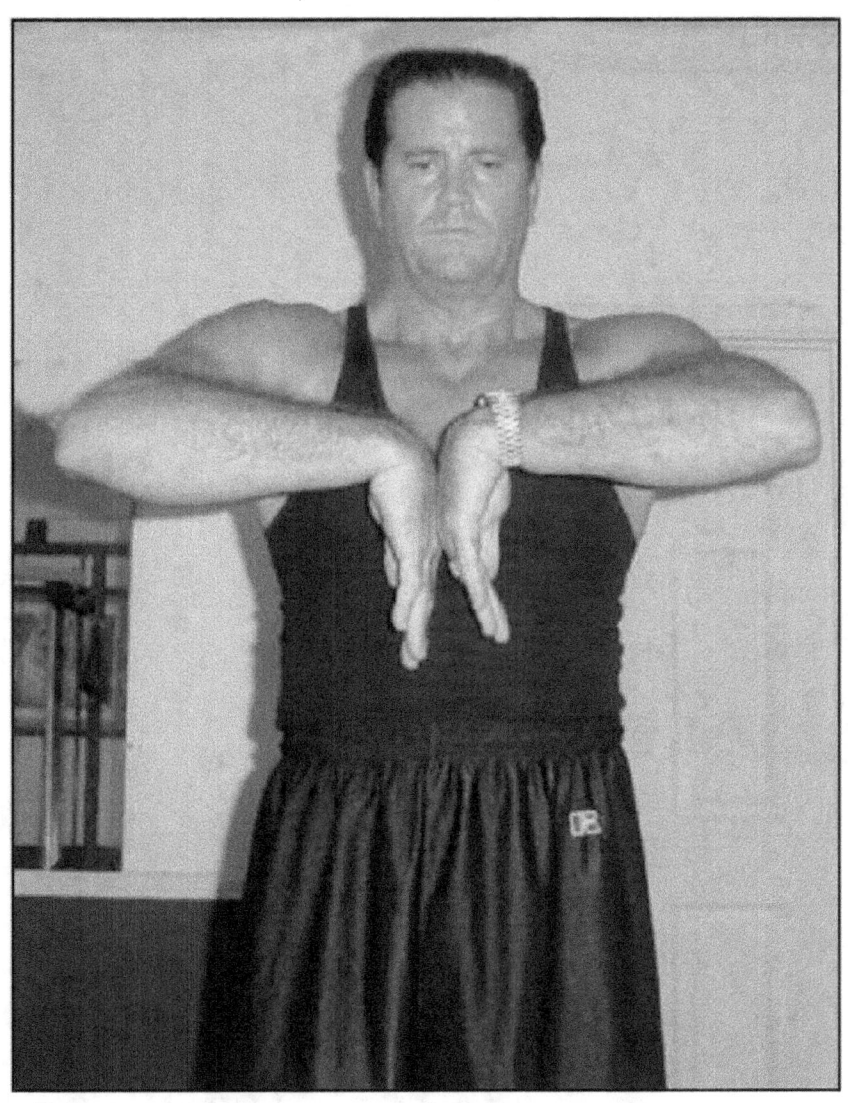

Take the wrists and press them against each other backwards.

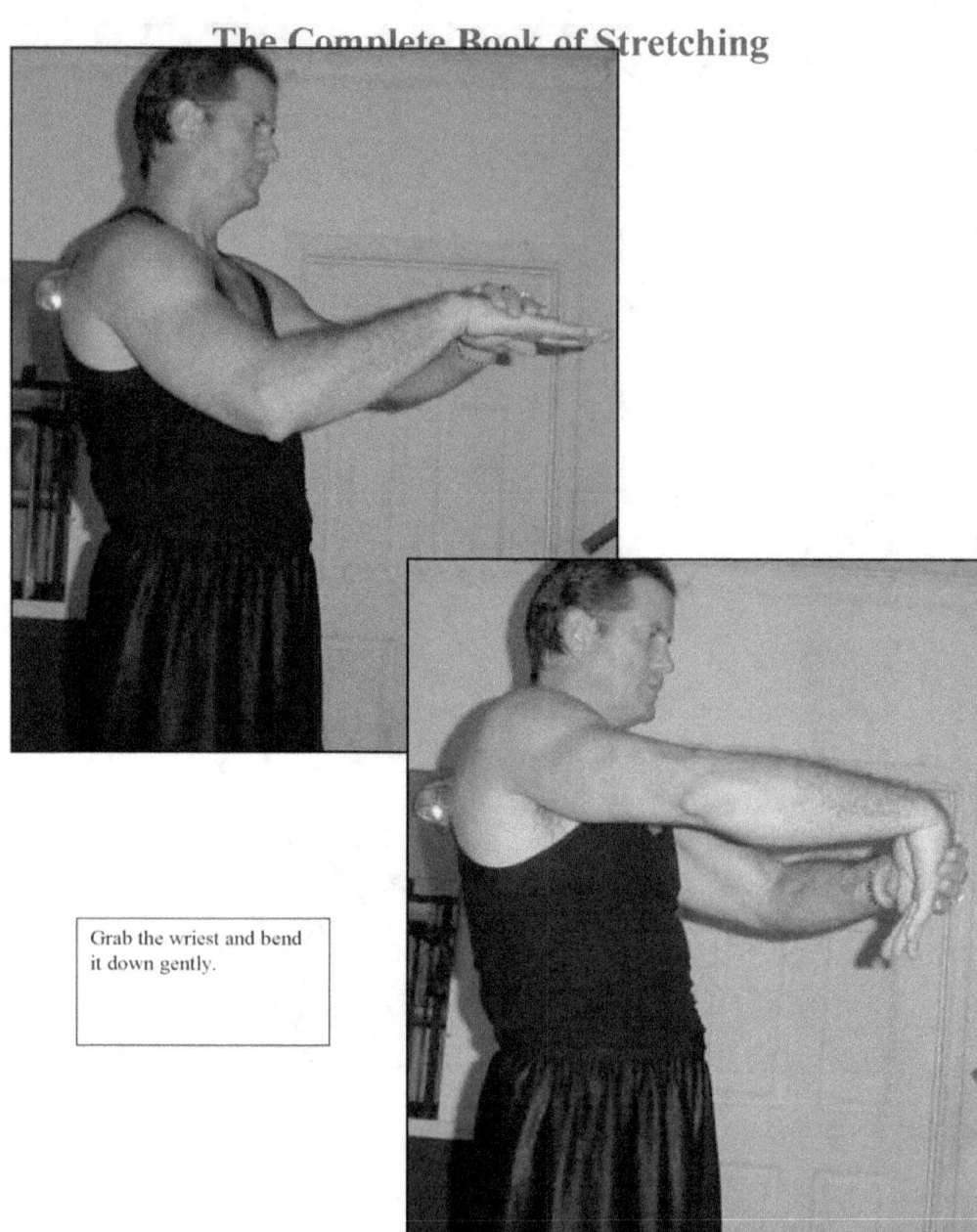

Grab the wriest and bend
it down gently.

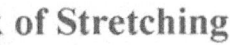

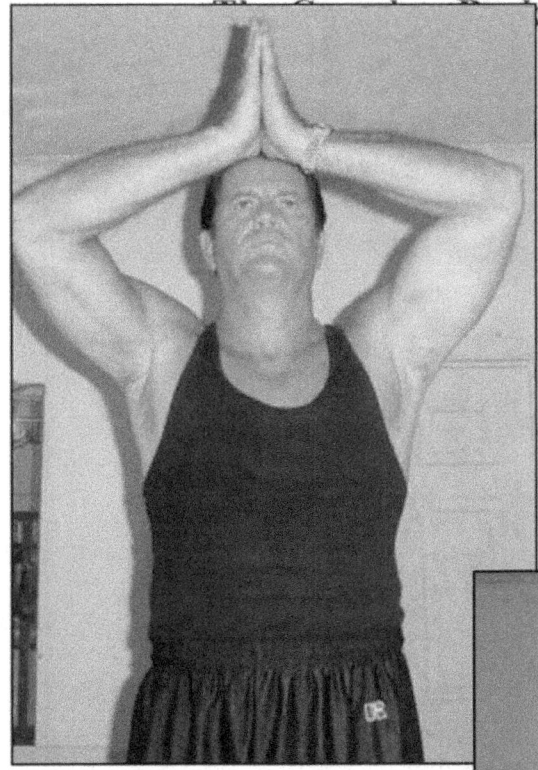

Start with the wrist up high in front of the body then bring them down to the chest.

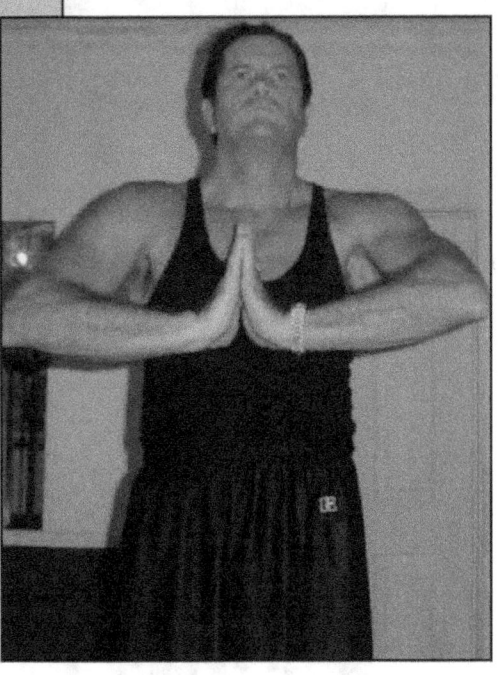

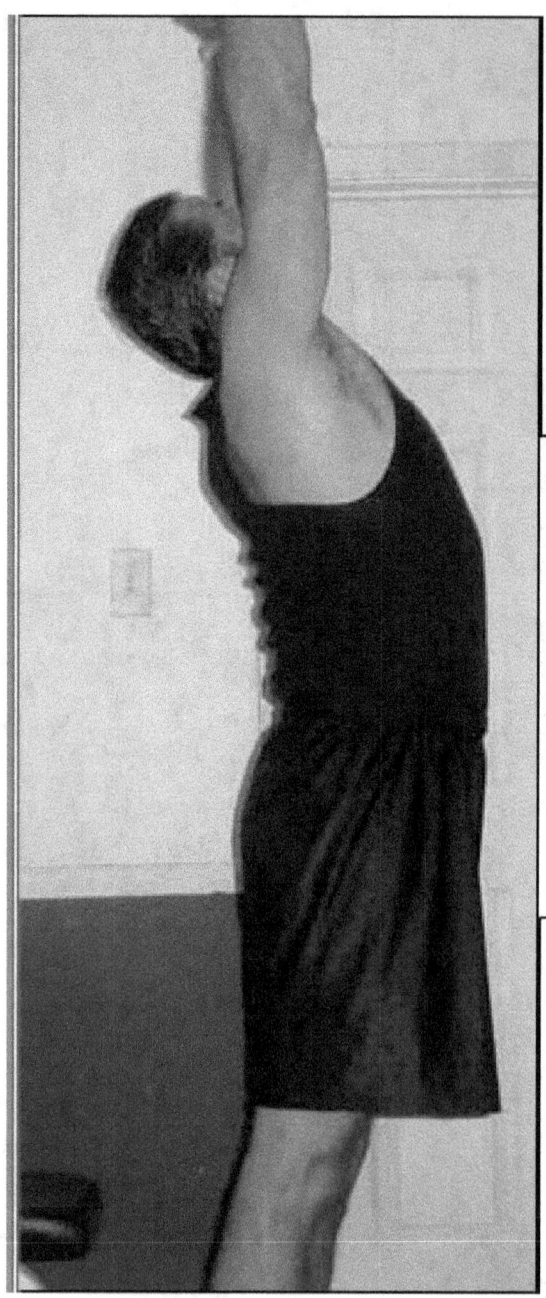

Stand very tall
and reach up,
then stretch up
to the toes
while reaching
as high as you
can.

Back Stretches

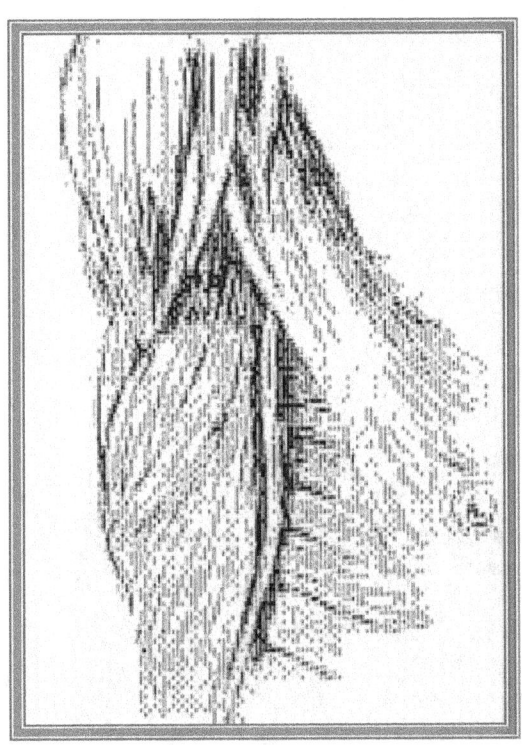

Do all stretches 6 to 8 times. Relax and breath easy, do not bounce or force the stretch..

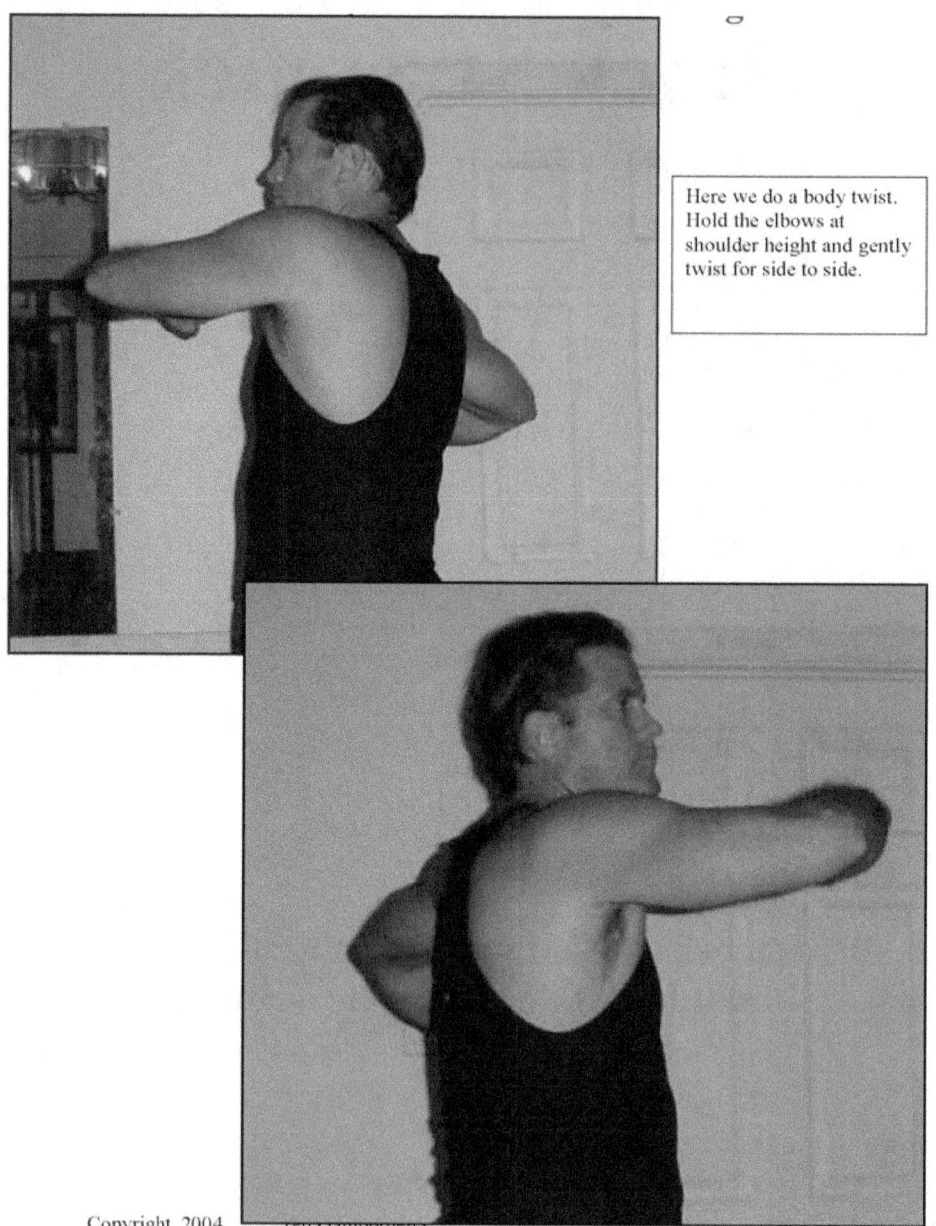

Here we do a body twist. Hold the elbows at shoulder height and gently twist for side to side.

This is a pelvic/back stretch. Hold onto a support and force the hips forward for the stretch.

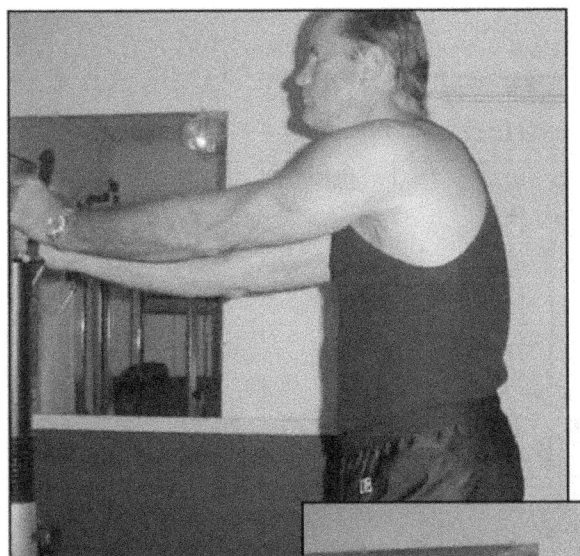

This is a pelvic/back stretch. Hold onto a support and force the hips forward for the stretch.

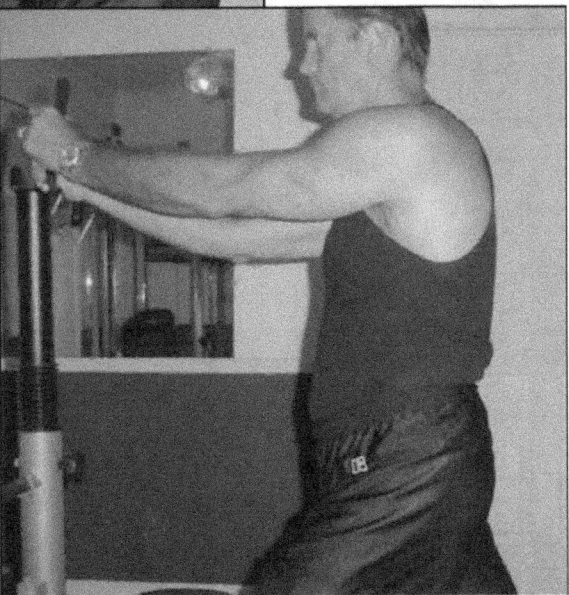

Here we loosen the back and hips by holding our arms up at the shoulders and twisting the body to the right and left..

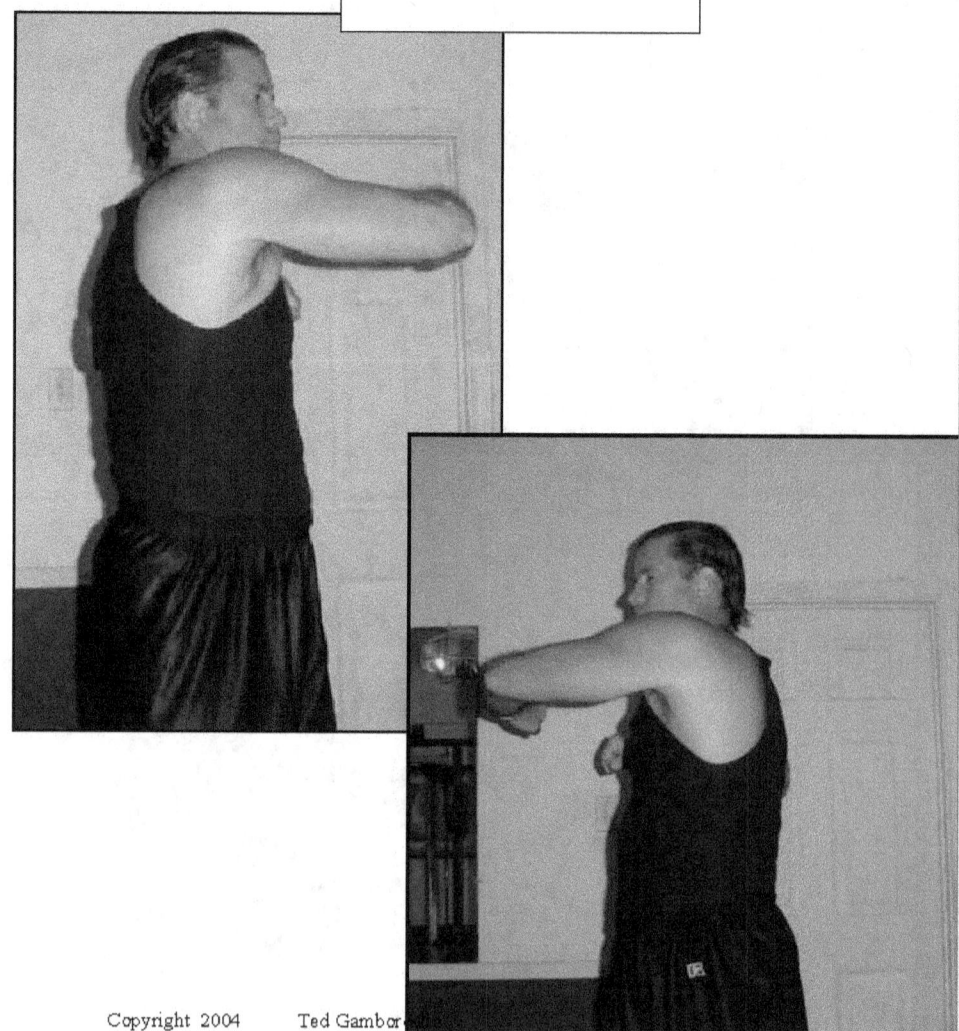

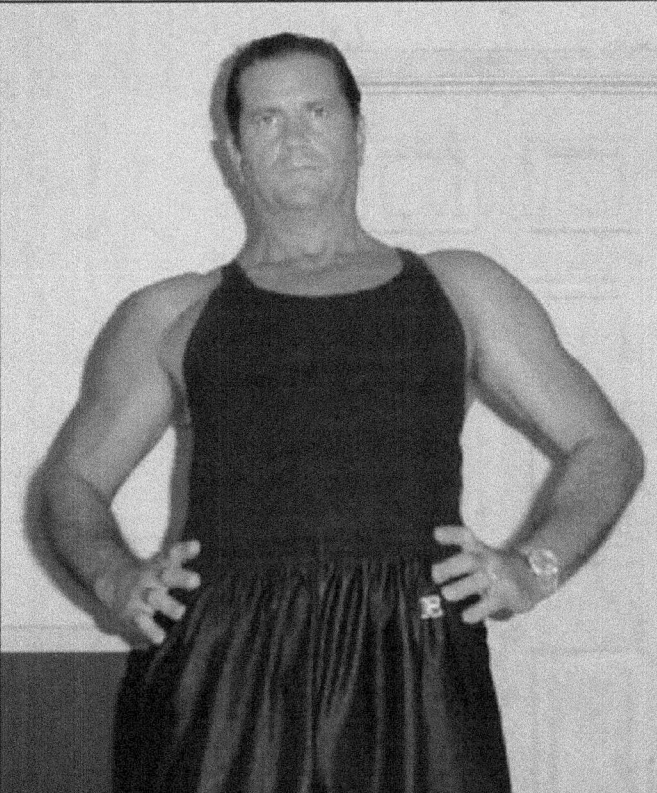

Here we do hip c
Hold the arms or
and rotate the bo
in gentle circles
and right.

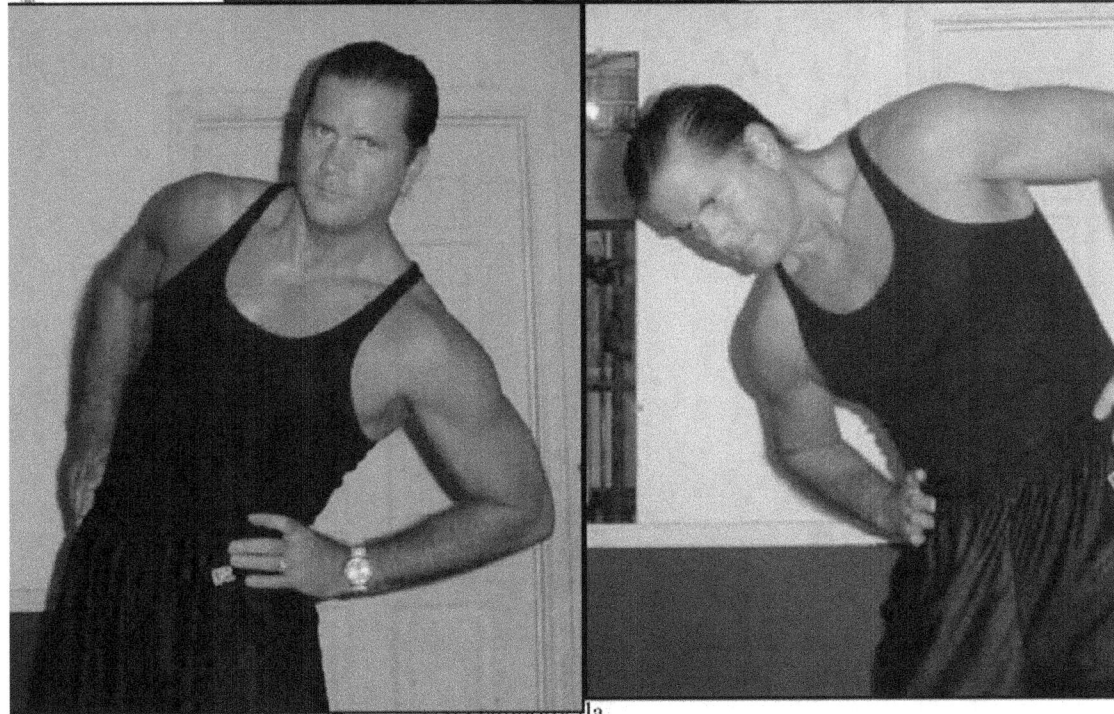

Reach up and grab the tricep of the opposite arm and pull it across the body.

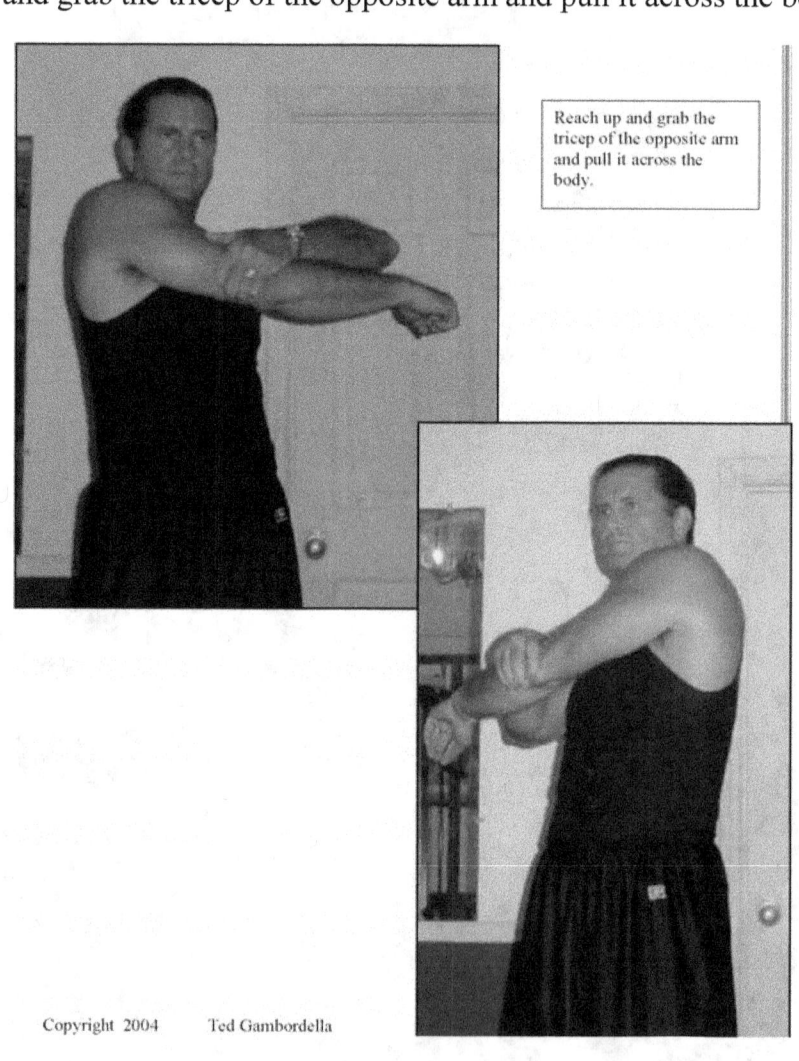

Reach up and grab the
tricep of the opposite arm
and pull it across the
body.

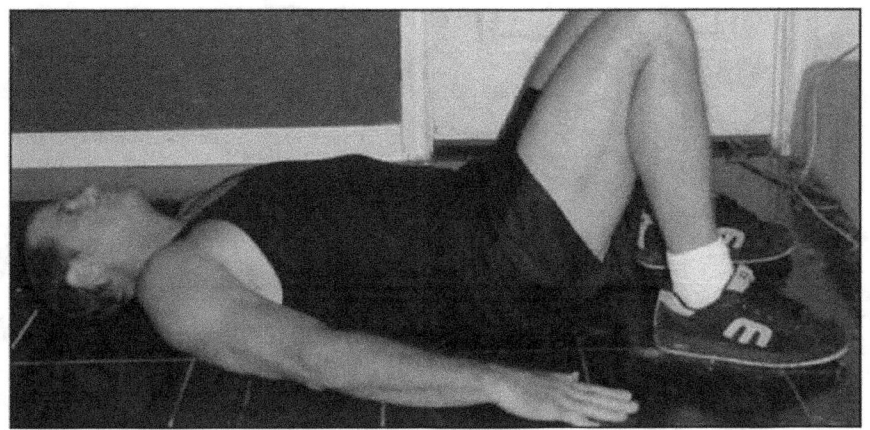

Here we loosen the back by lying with the arms directly to the sides and then arching up our hips.

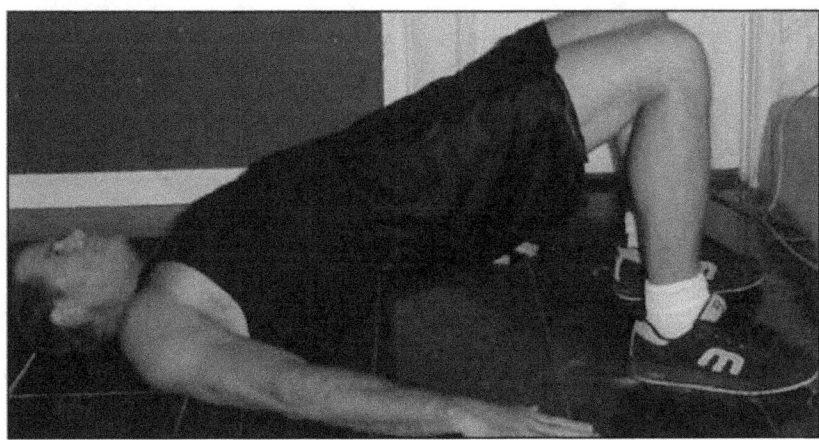

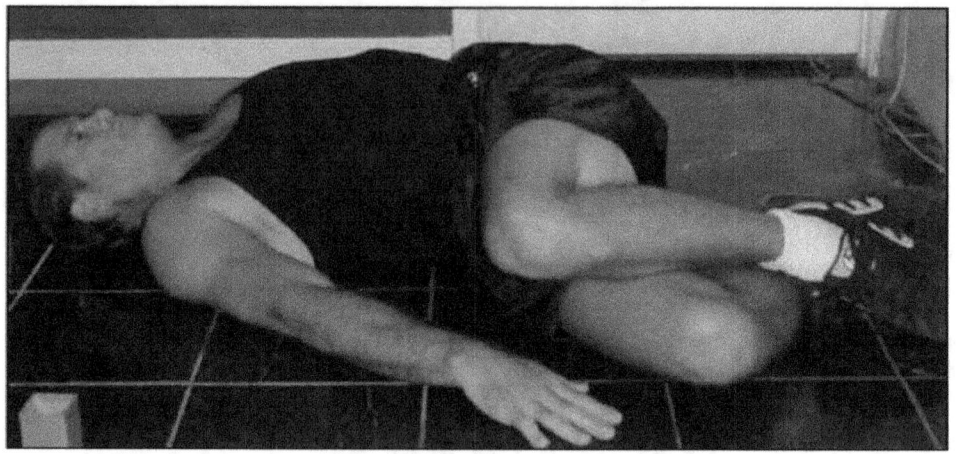

While lying on your back, keep the legs together and roll them from side to side.

Roll the body up over the hips and try to touch the knees to the ground on the sides of your head.

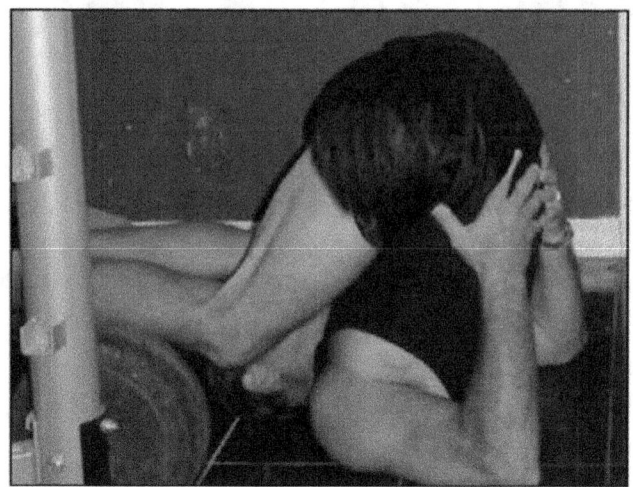

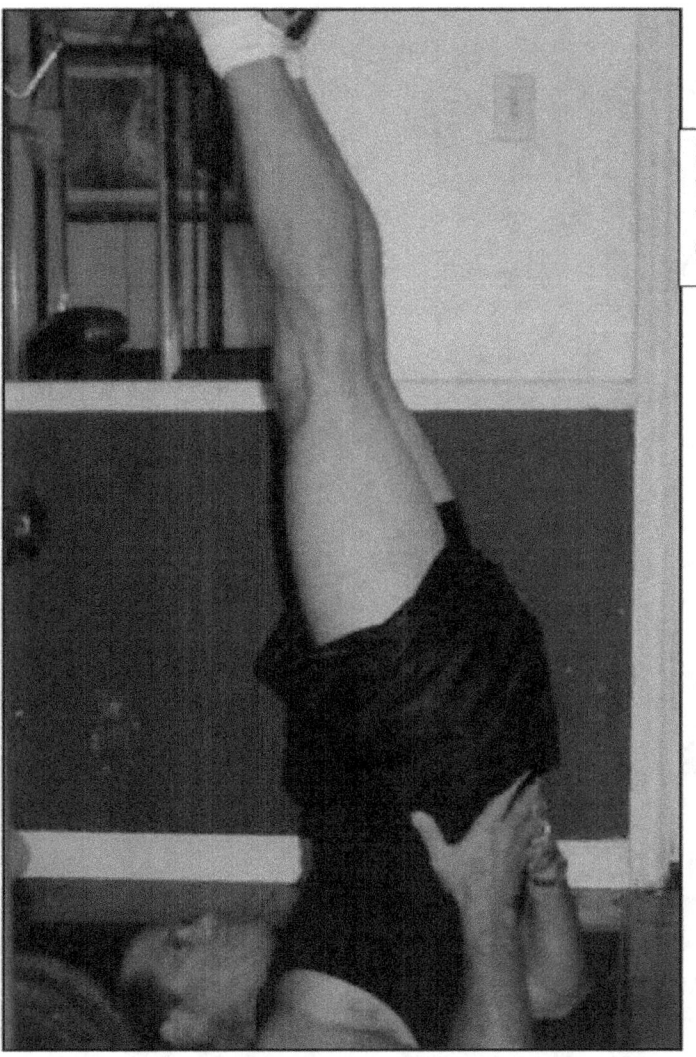

Here we support the body with the arms on the hips while forcing the legs straight up.

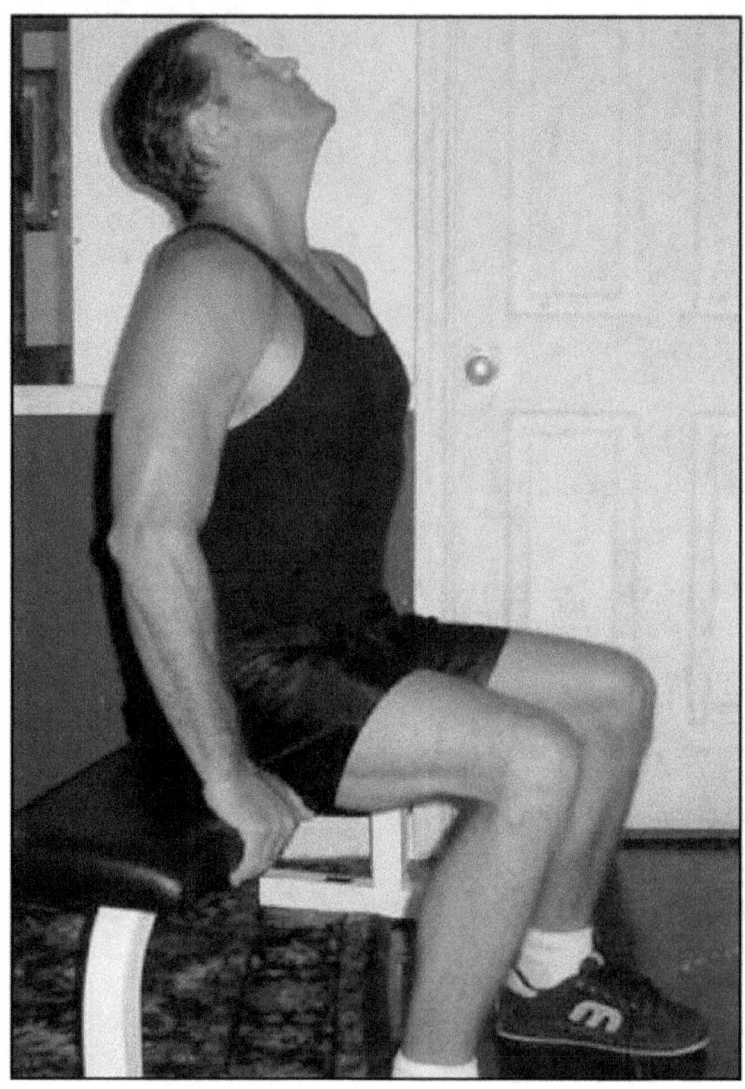

Sit on a bench or a chair and keeping the back straight pull the head and neck back as far a possible.

Hand the body over the edge of a bench, letting the neck relax and stretch. Keep the hands behind the back Place the arms on the bench and lean the body up into a stretched position, and then back down to rest on the elbows.

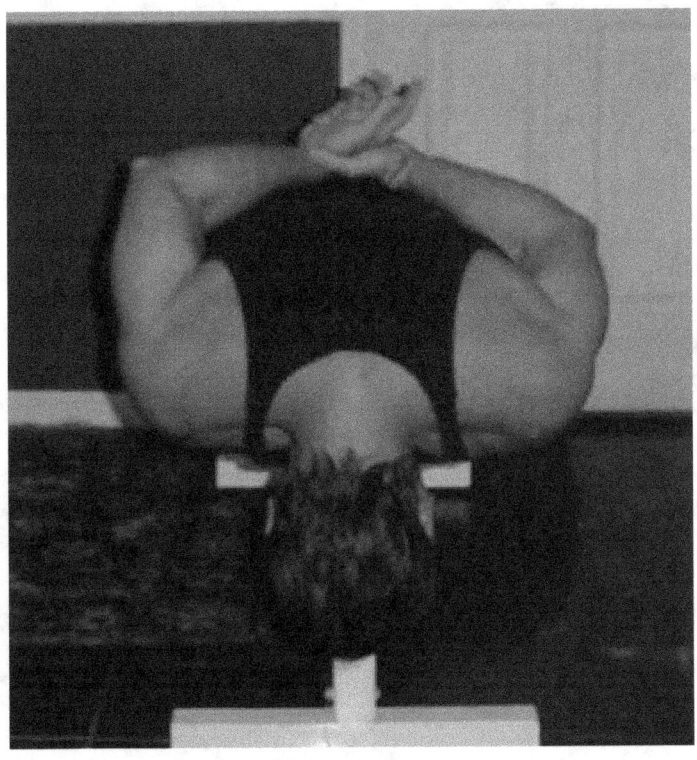

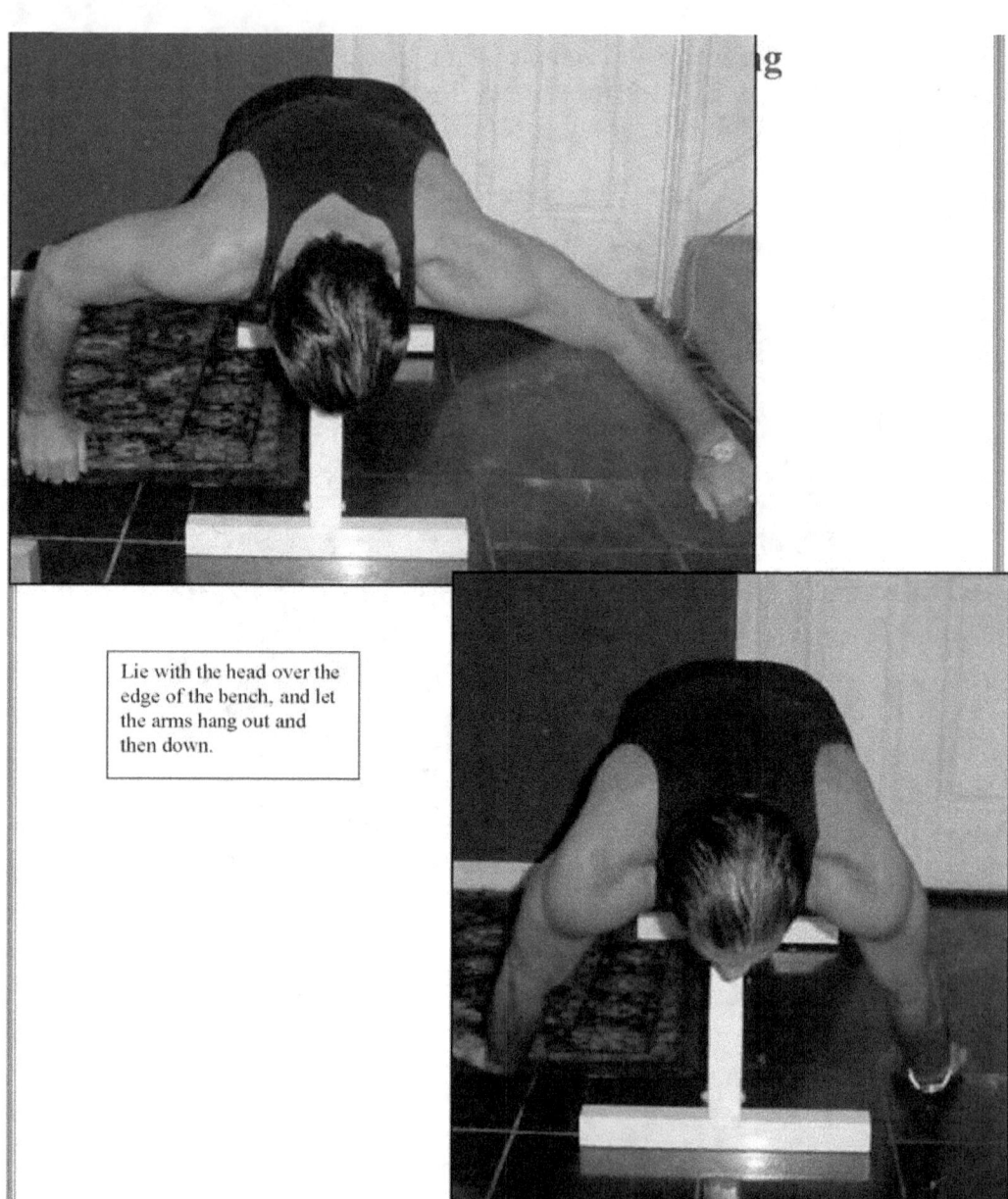

Lie with the head over the
edge of the bench, and let
the arms hang out and
then down.

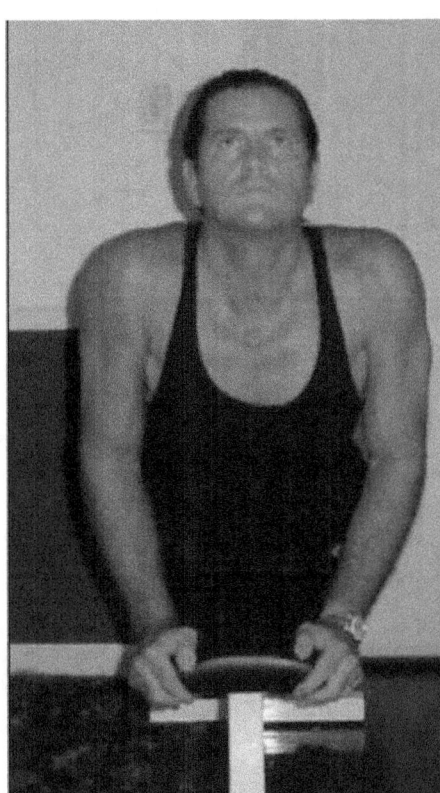

Place the arms on the bench and lean the body up into a stretched position, and then back down to rest on the elbows.

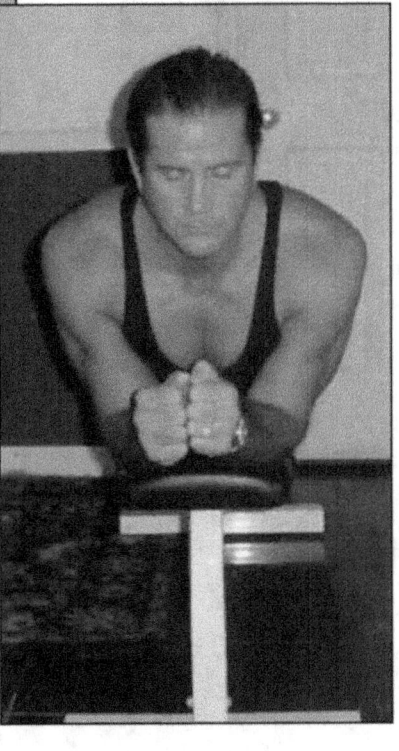

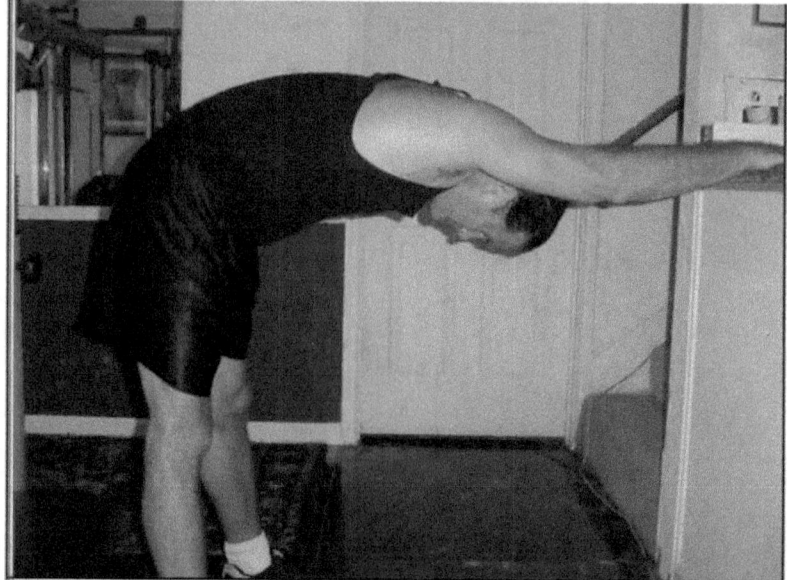

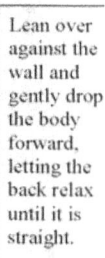

Lean over against the wall and gently drop the body forward, letting the back relax until it is straight.

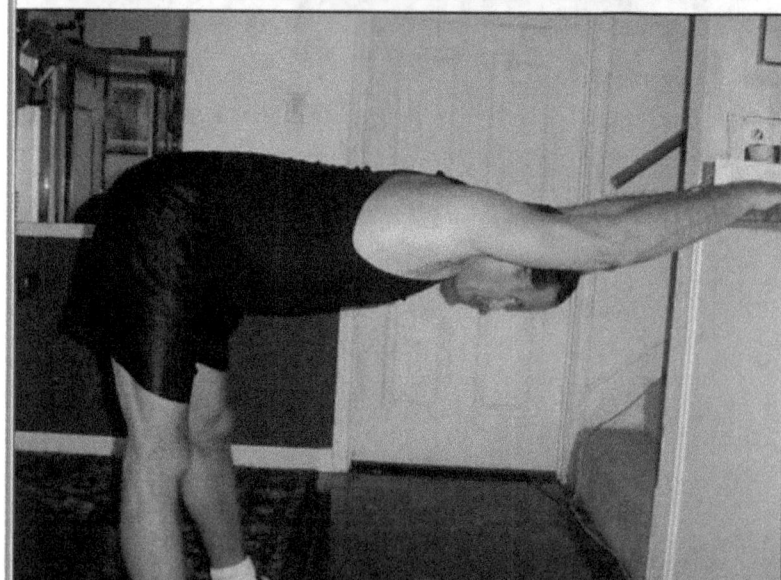

Sit on the bench and place one arm on the hip, then gently turn to the right and left. Use the other arm to press on the knee for more turn.

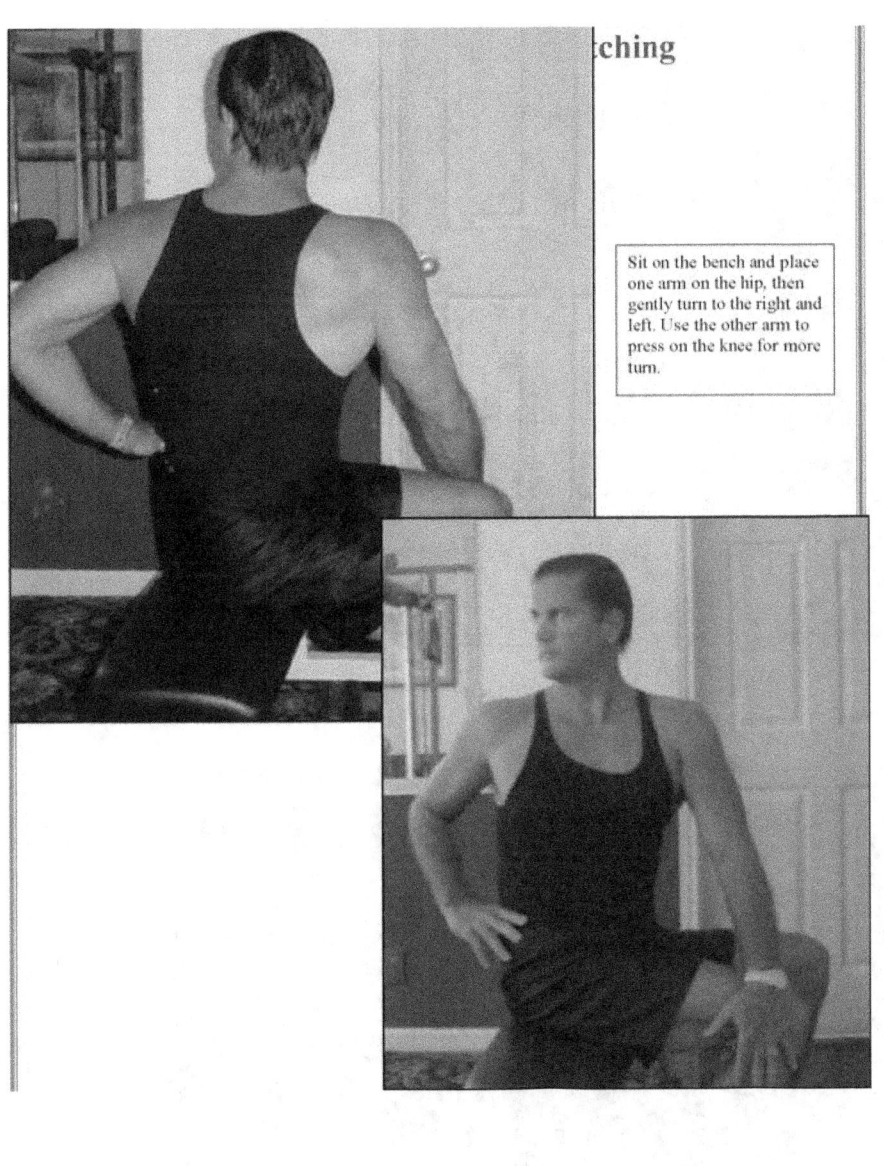

Sit on the bench and place one arm on the hip, then gently turn to the right and left. Use the other arm to press on the knee for more turn.

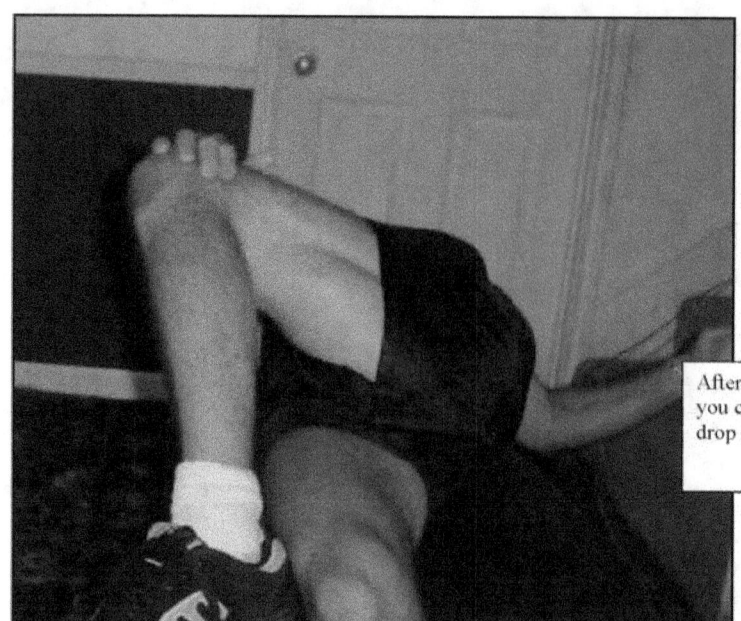

After you have relaxed you can hold the knee and drop it to each side.

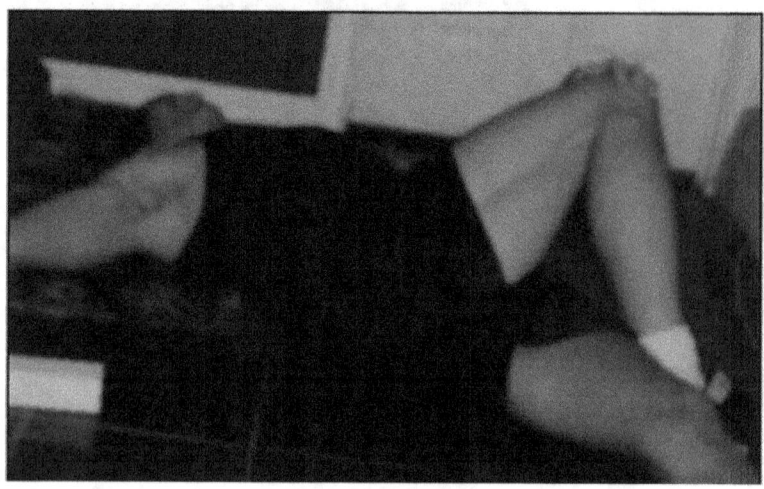

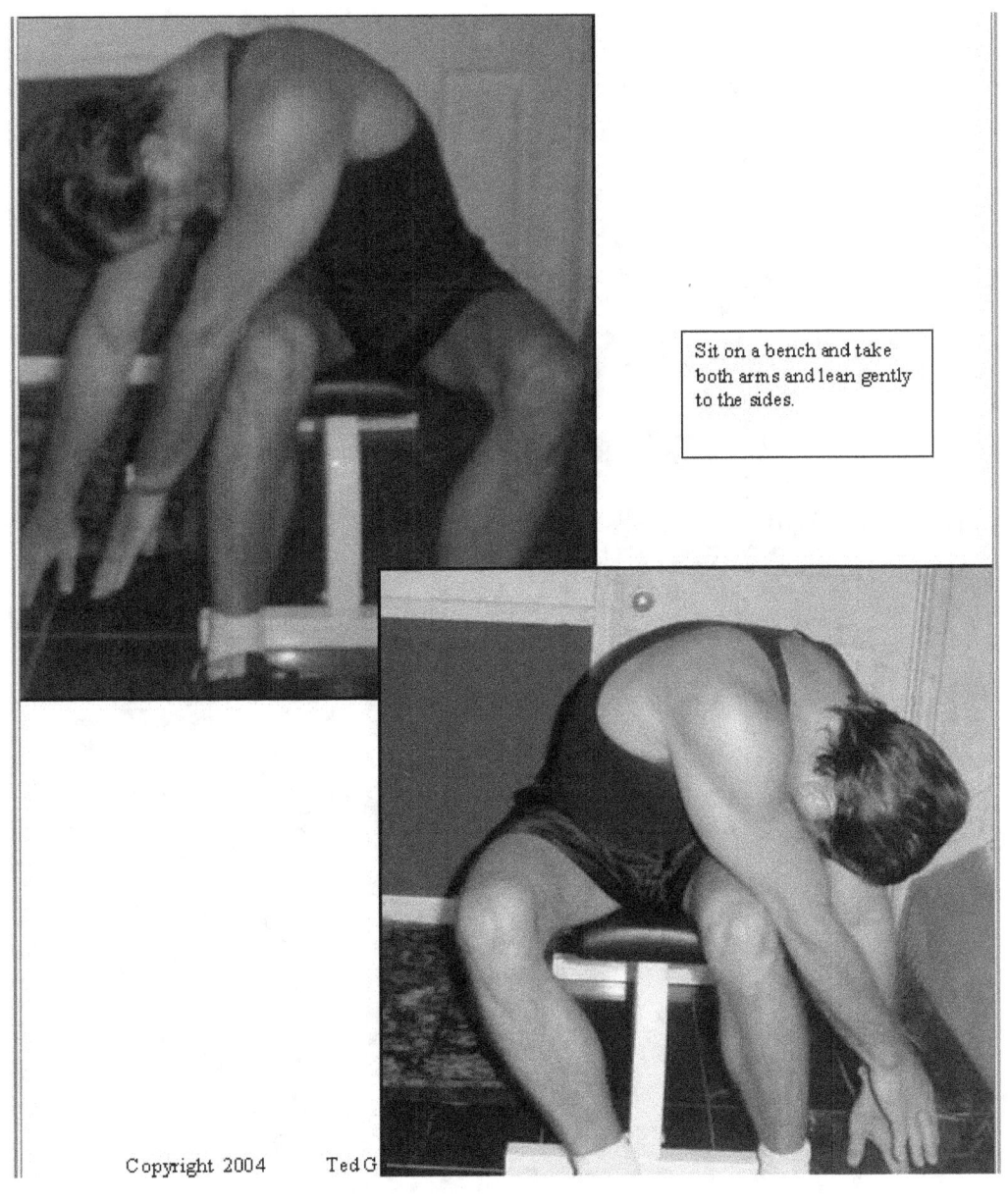

Sit on a bench and take both arms and lean gently to the sides.

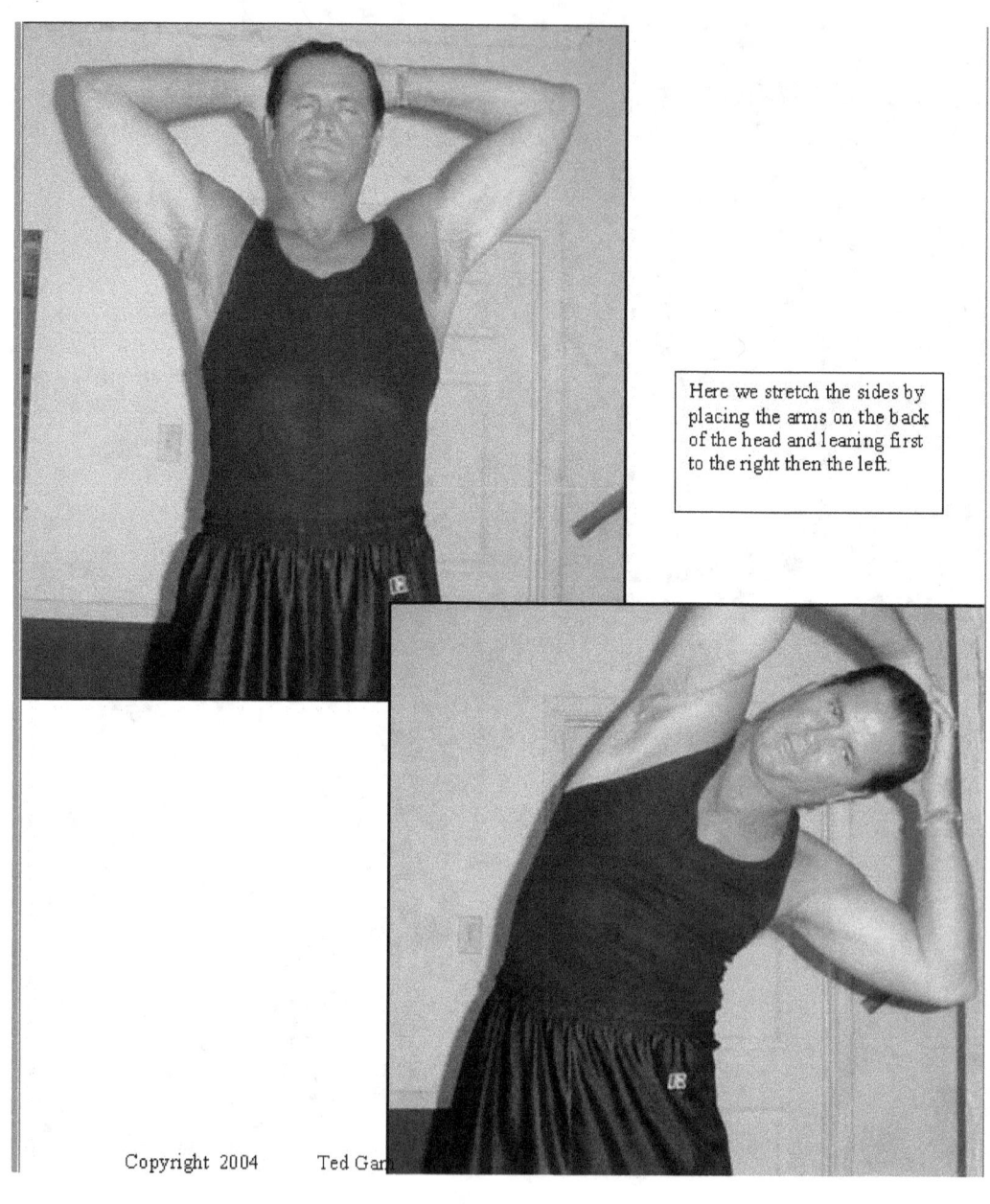

Here we stretch the sides by placing the arms on the back of the head and leaning first to the right then the left.

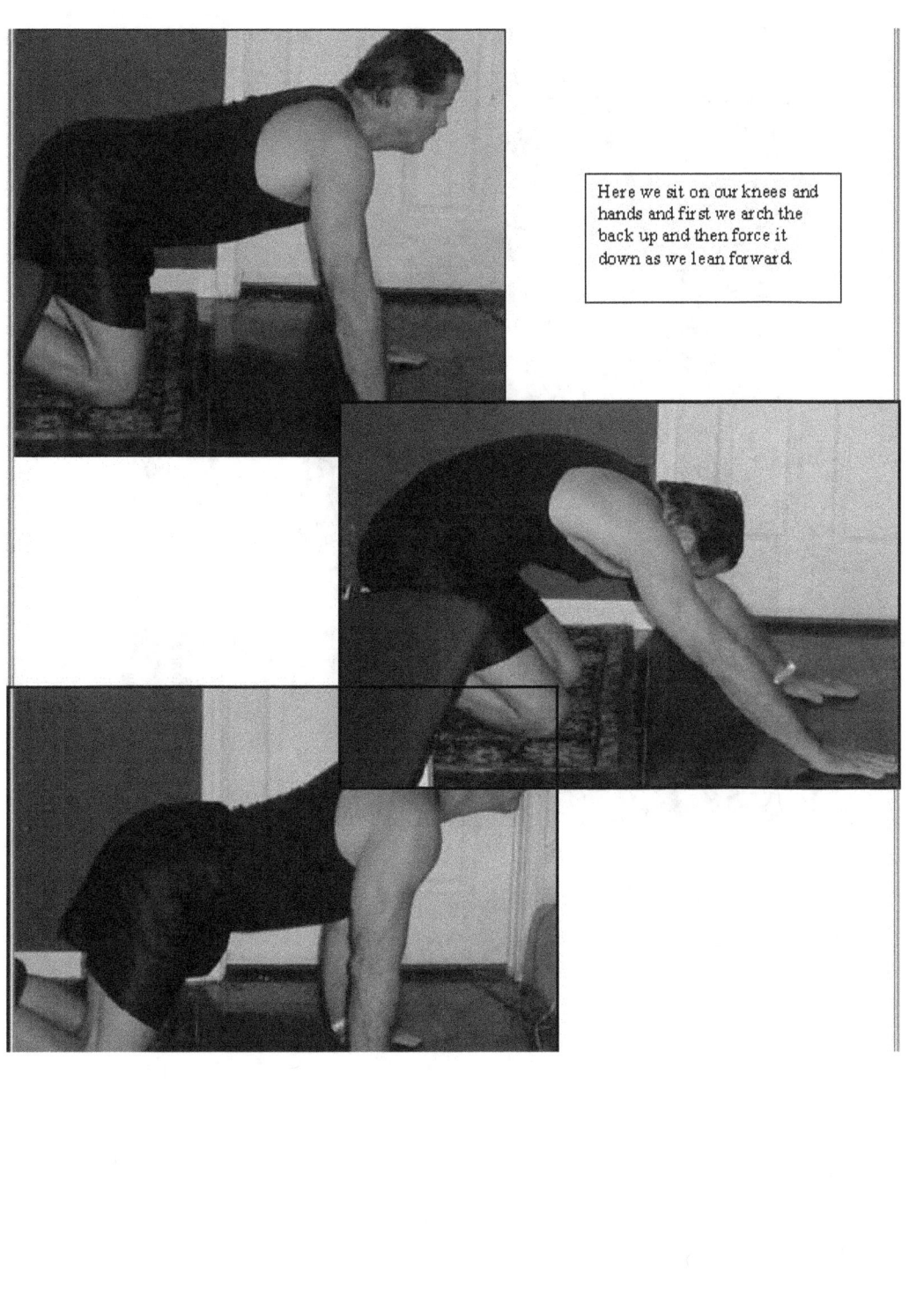

Here we sit on our knees and hands and first we arch the back up and then force it down as we lean forward.

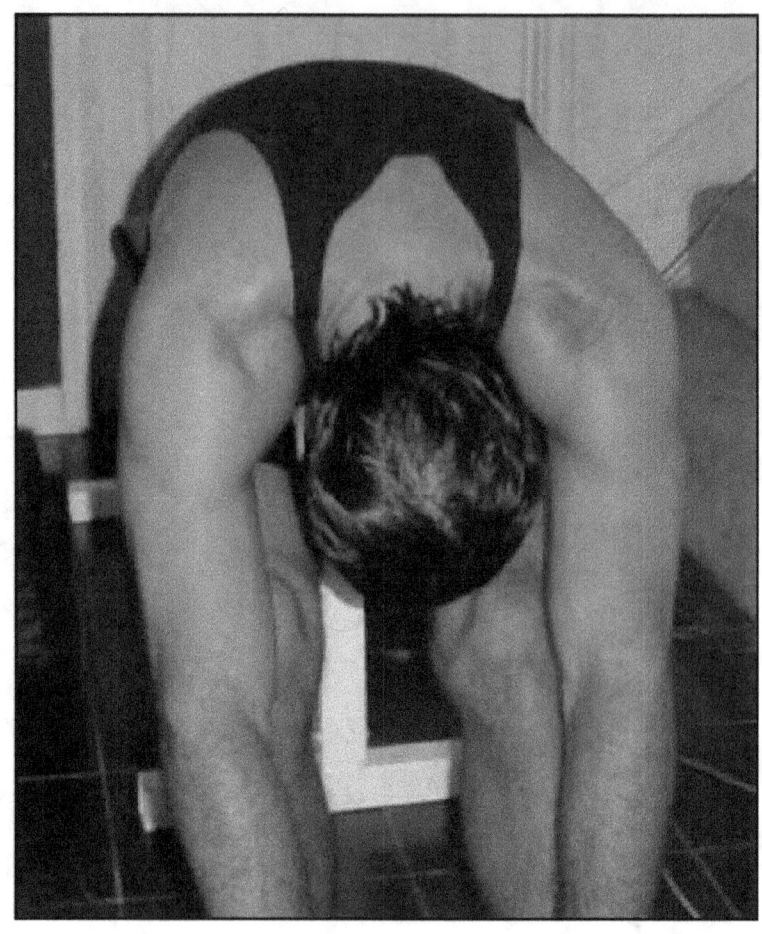

You can relax in a chair by leaning forward and letting the arms drop.

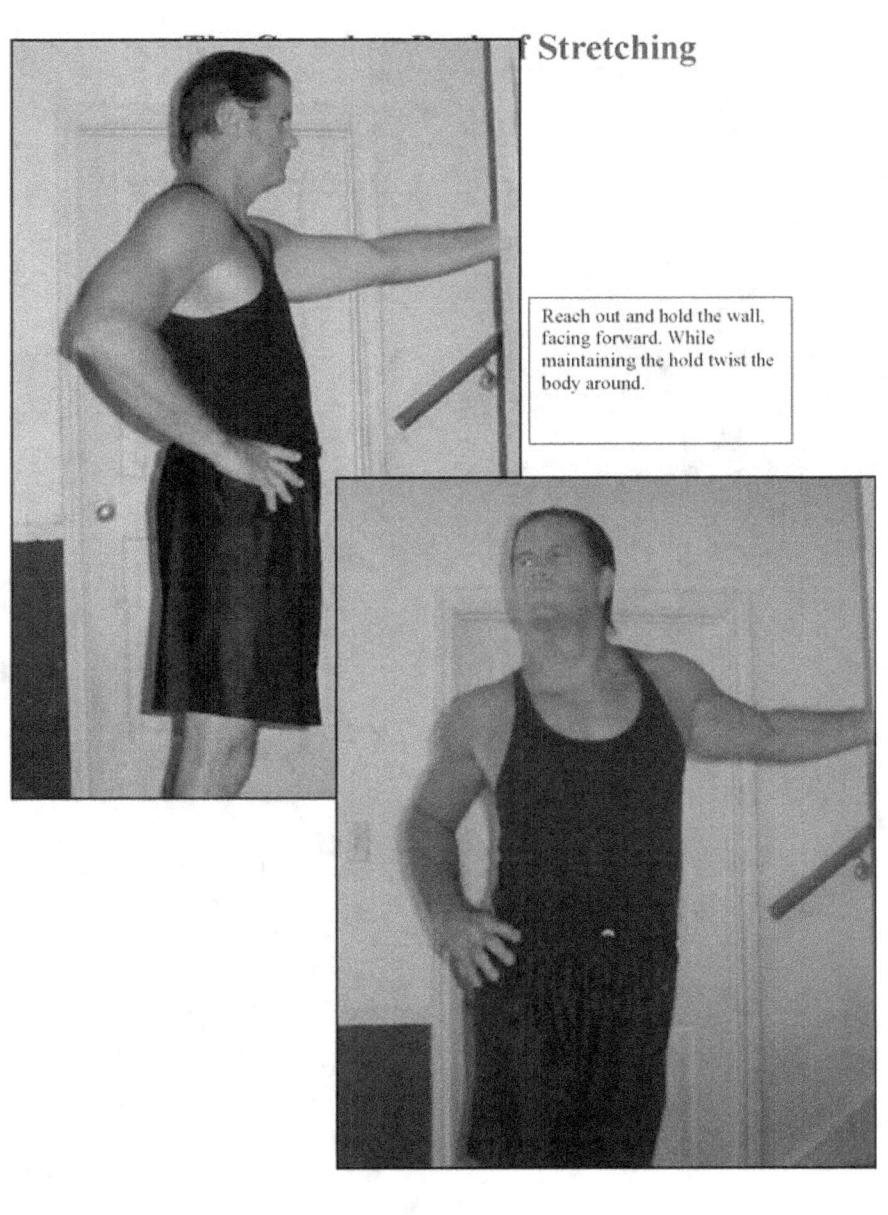

Reach out and hold the wall, facing forward. While maintaining the hold twist the body around.

Sit on the ground and cross the legs, holding onto the knee and gently turning the

Sit on the ground and cross the legs, holding onto the knee and gently turning the body.

body.

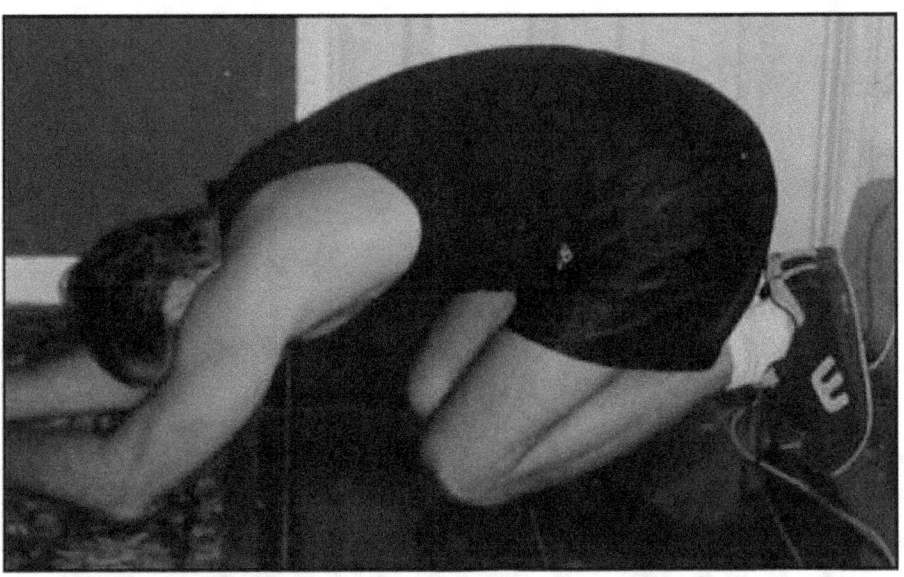

This is a simple Cat stretch. You are on your hands a knees and you flex your back up like a cat

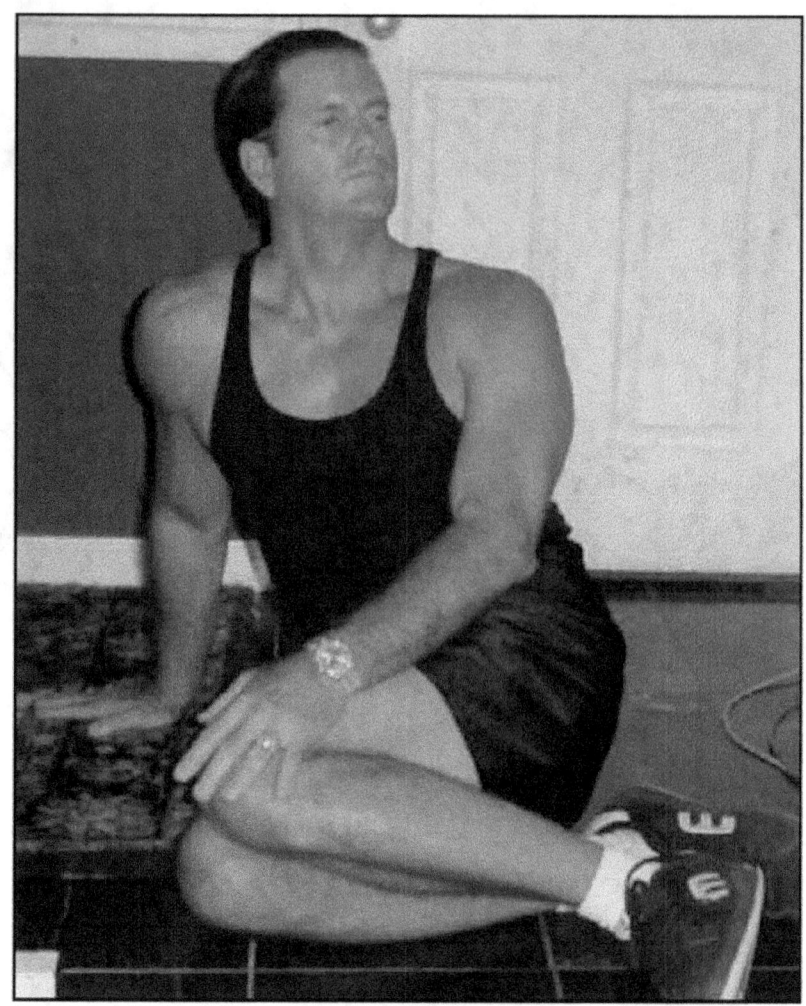

Sit on the floor and drop the knees to the side and turn the body in the opposite direction while pushing down on the knees.

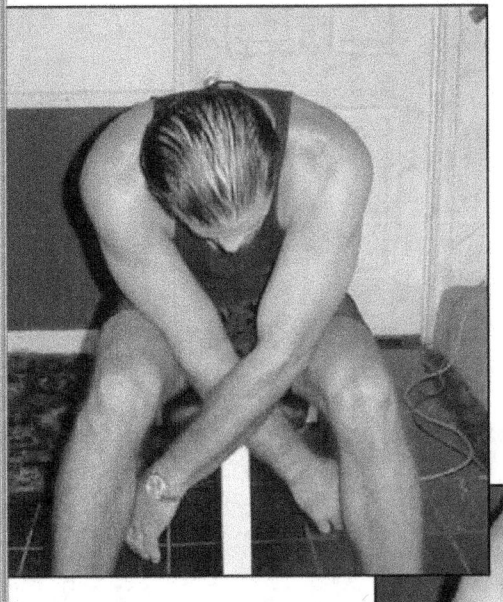

Sit on the bench and cross the arms in front of the body then lean forward and drop the arms to the toes.

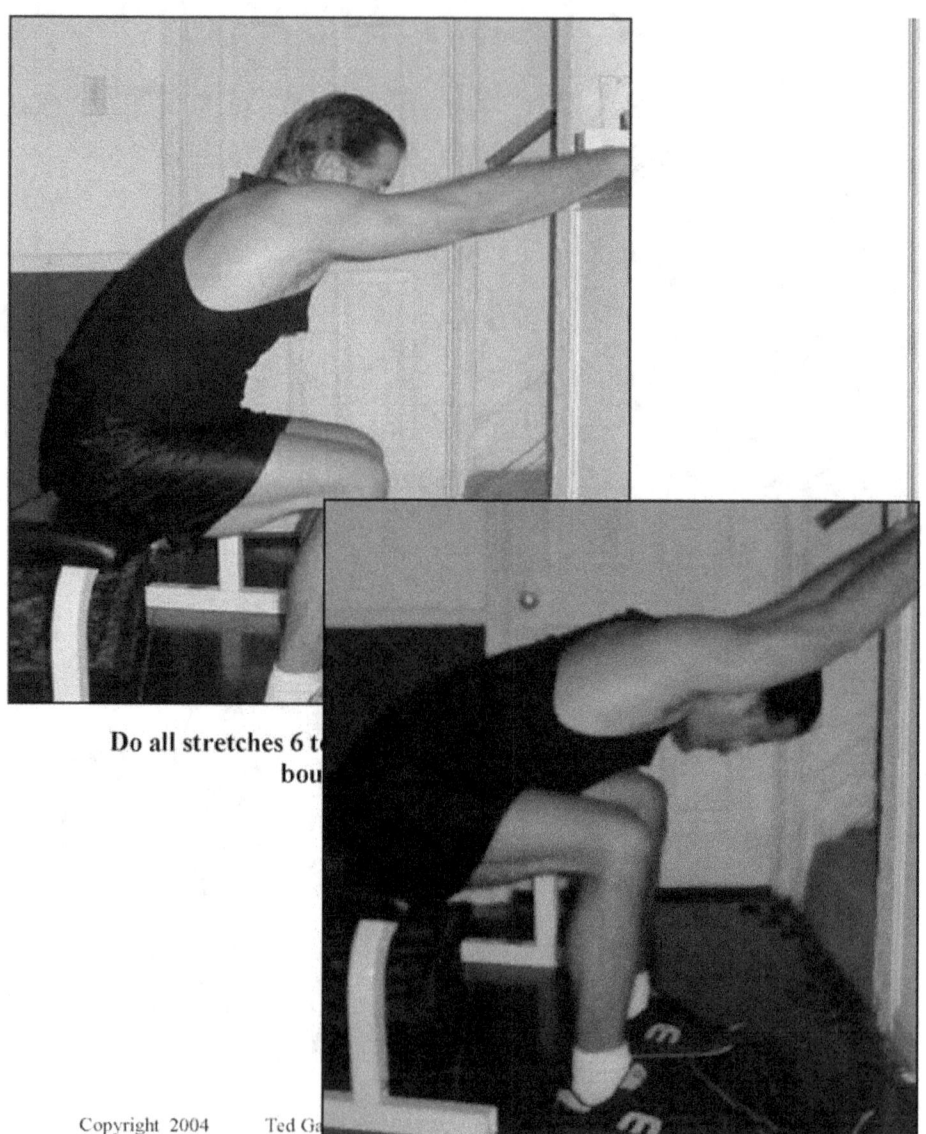

Do all stretches 6 t...
bou...

Hold onto a bar or the wall and stand tall, now drop a leg back and lean forward to stretch the hamstrings.

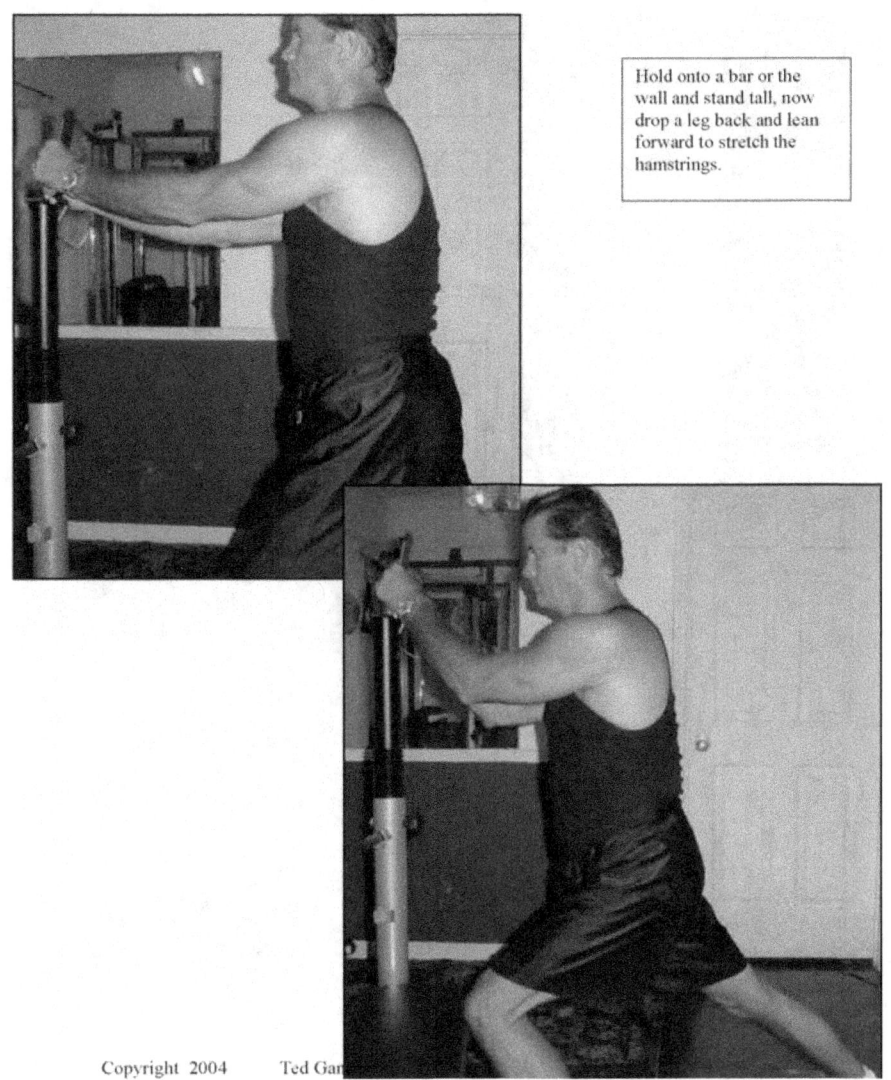

Hold onto a bar or the wall and stand tall, now drop a leg back and lean forward to stretch the hamstrings.

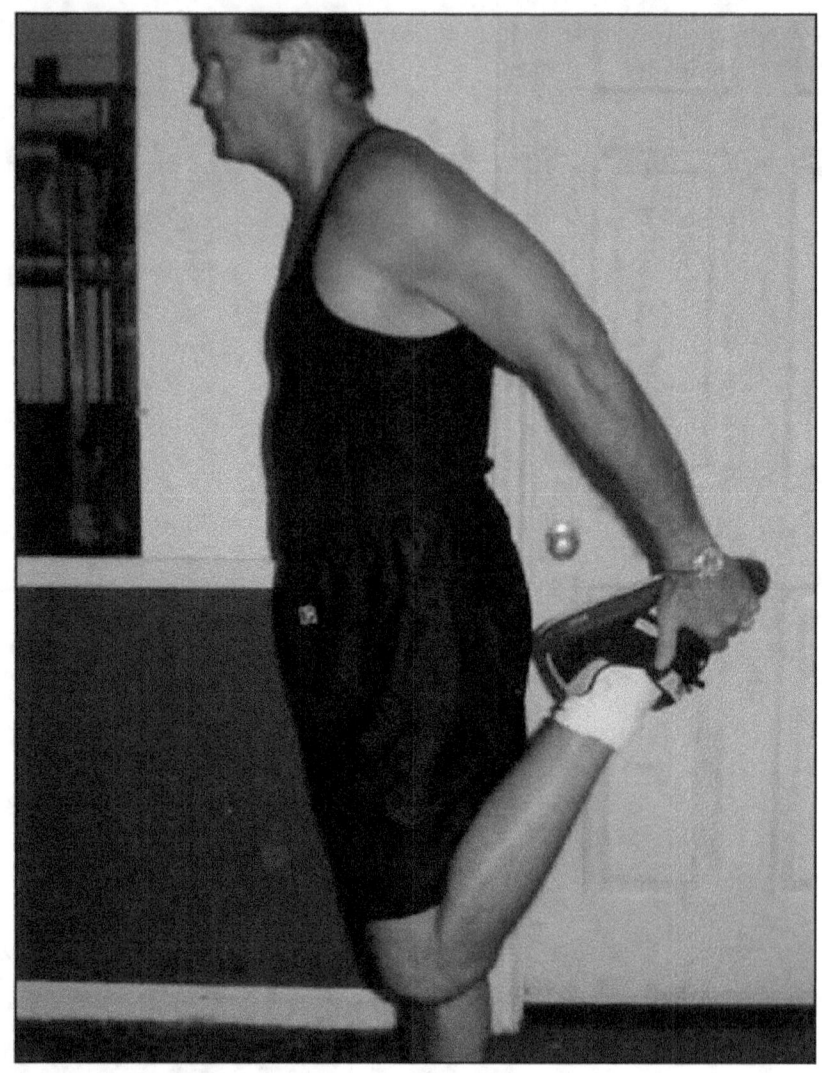

Stand tall and reach back and grab the foot, pulling it up to the buttocks.

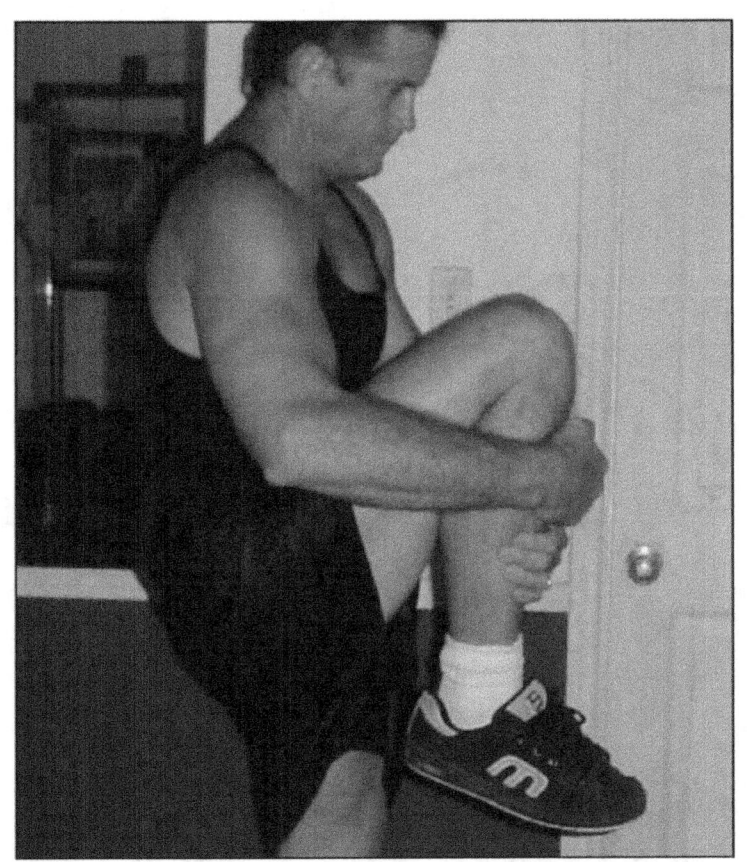

Stand tall and reach down to grab the knee, pull it up into the chest.

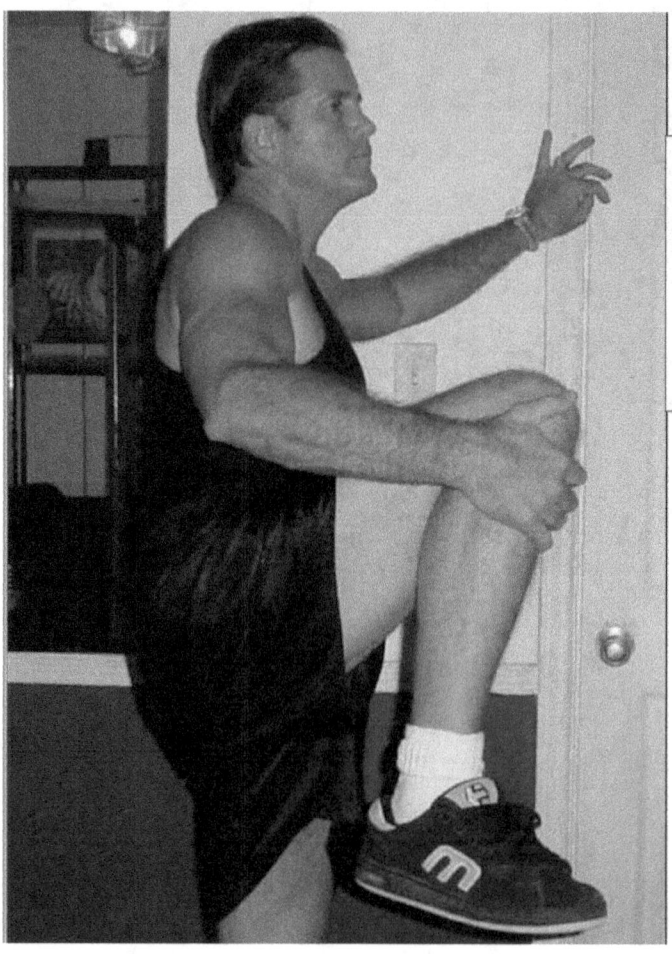

Lean against a wall for support. Reach down and grab the knee and lift it high to the front of your body.

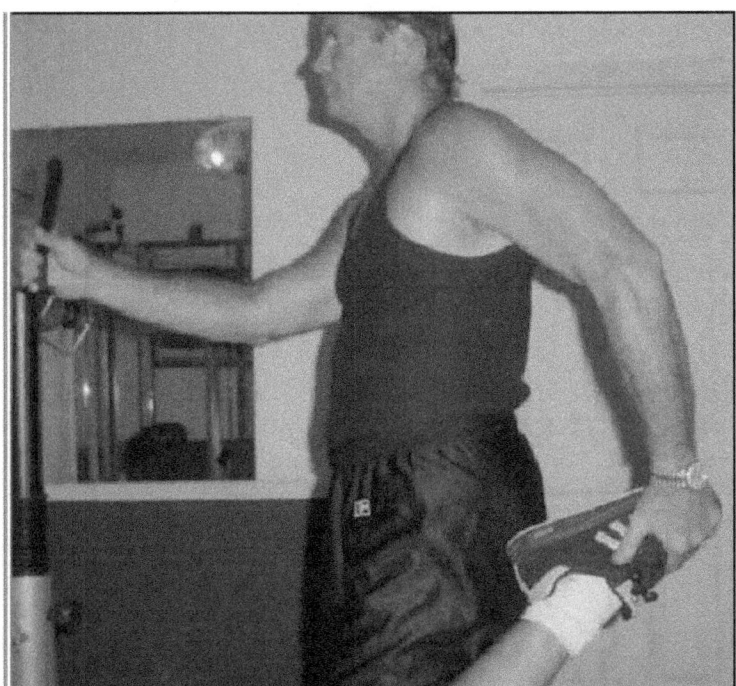

Hold on to a support and reach back to grab the foot, now lean over and pull up gently on the leg. Repeat to both sides.

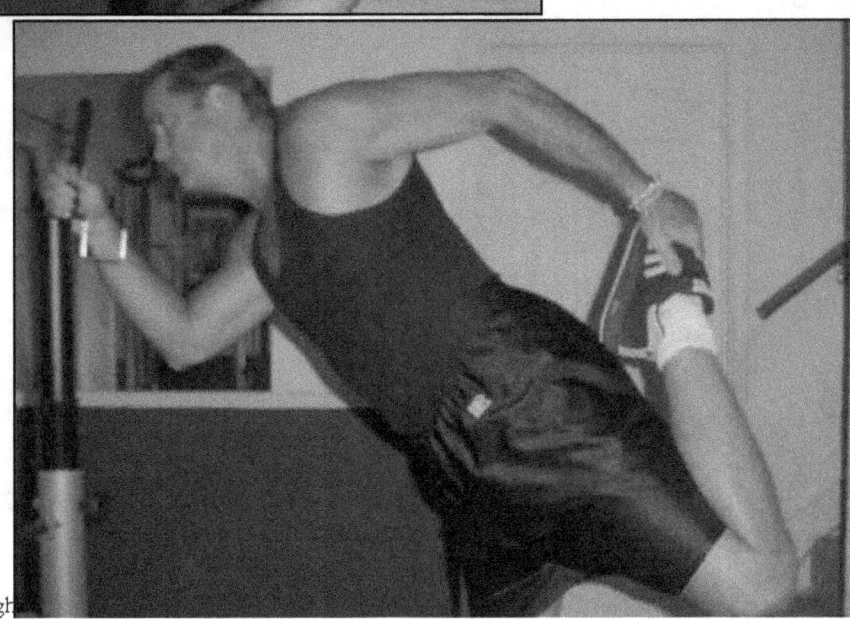

Hold the knee high to the body and then slowly turn the leg and hip to the side. This is a great stretch for the hips. .

As a continuation of the hip stretch, you can pull the leg all the way around the body until it is at a right angle.

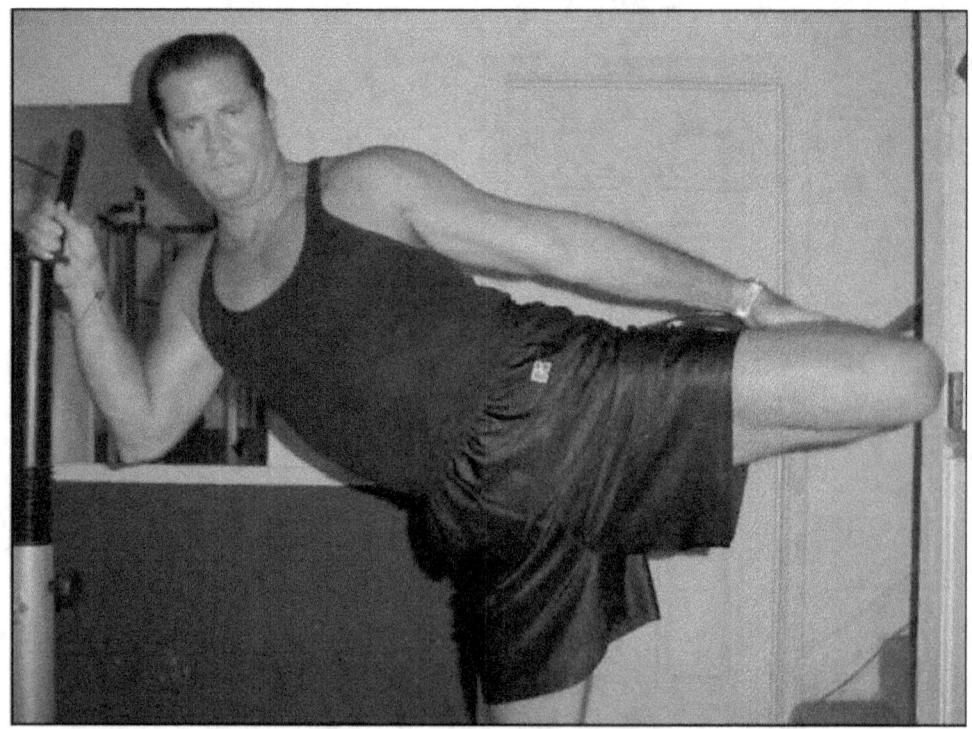

Here we hold the knee high and bring the leg around in a circle all the way to so that the foot faces backwards.

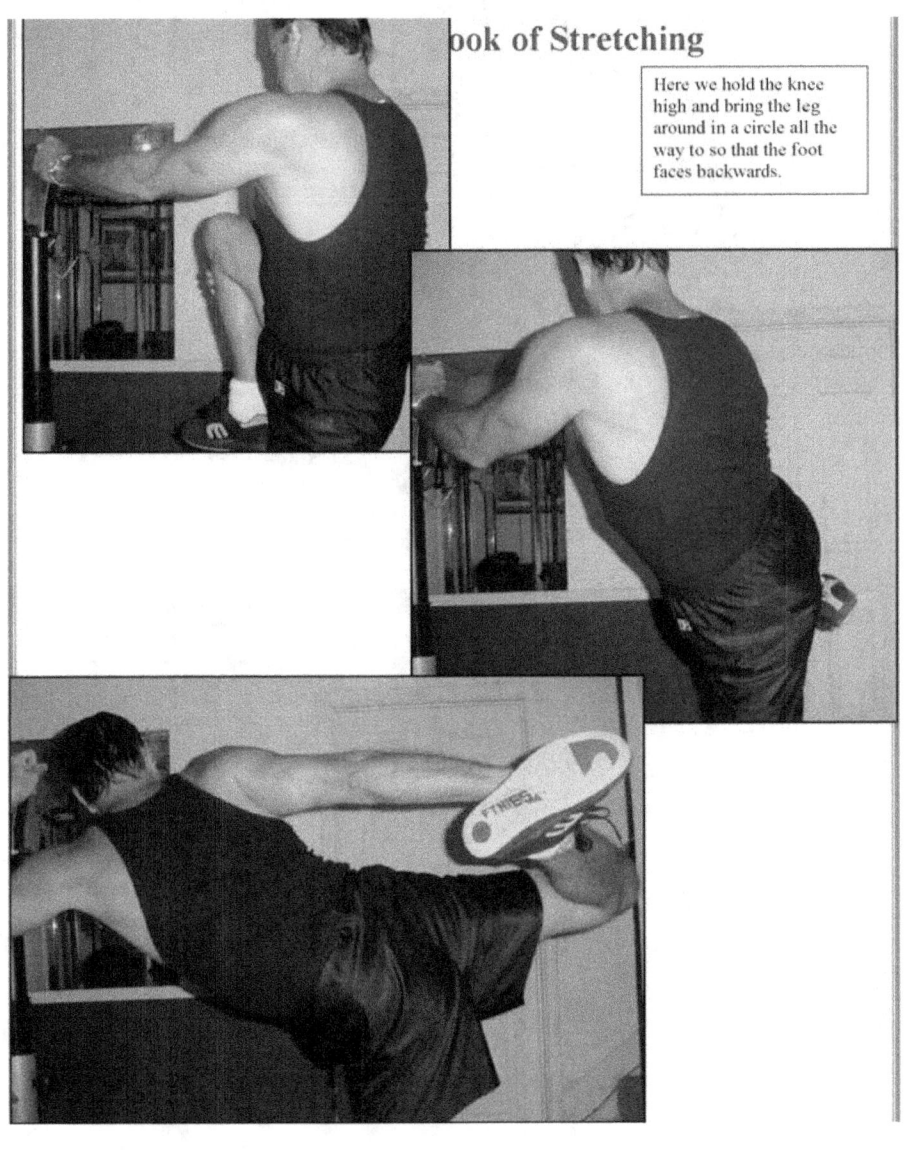

ook of Stretching

Here we hold the knee high and bring the leg around in a circle all the way to so that the foot faces backwards.

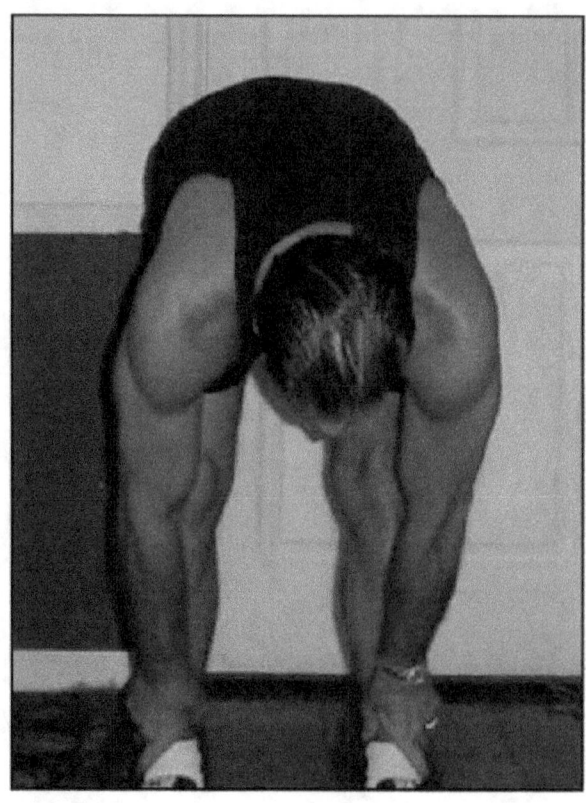

Lean over and let the body relax, try to touch the fingers to the ground.

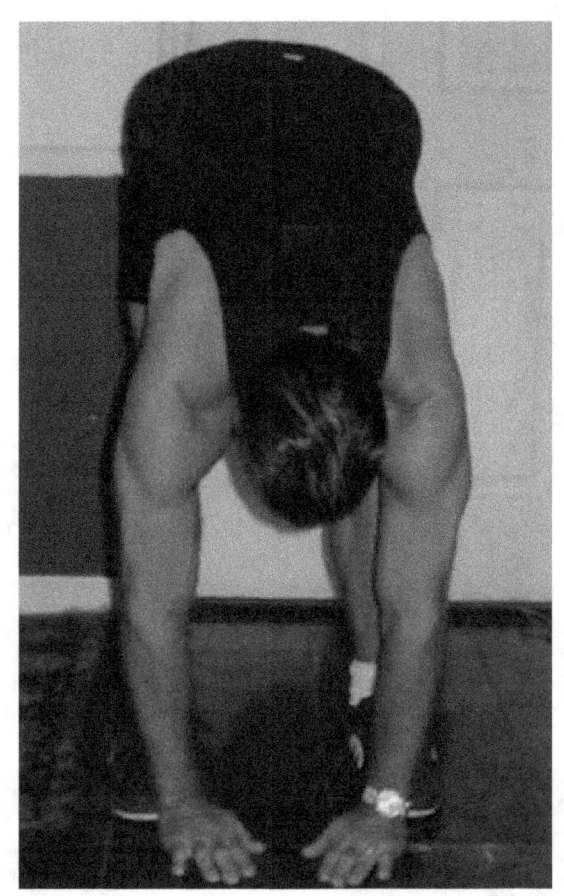

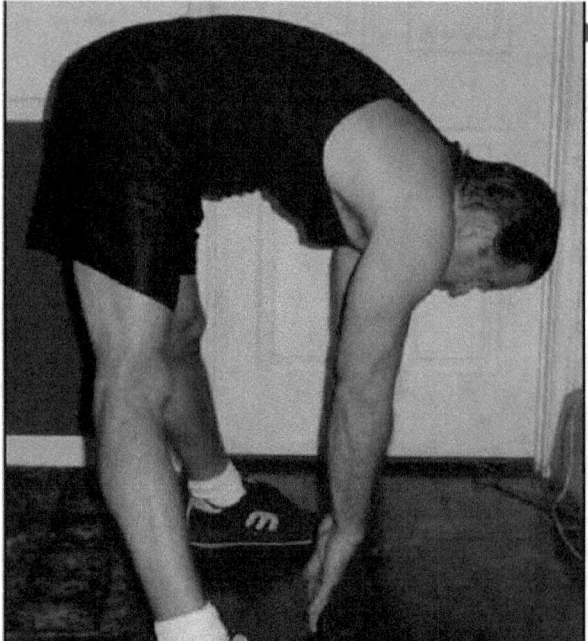

Here we le
a step reac
further bac
step.

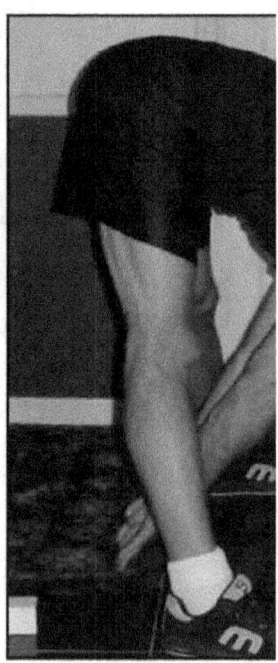

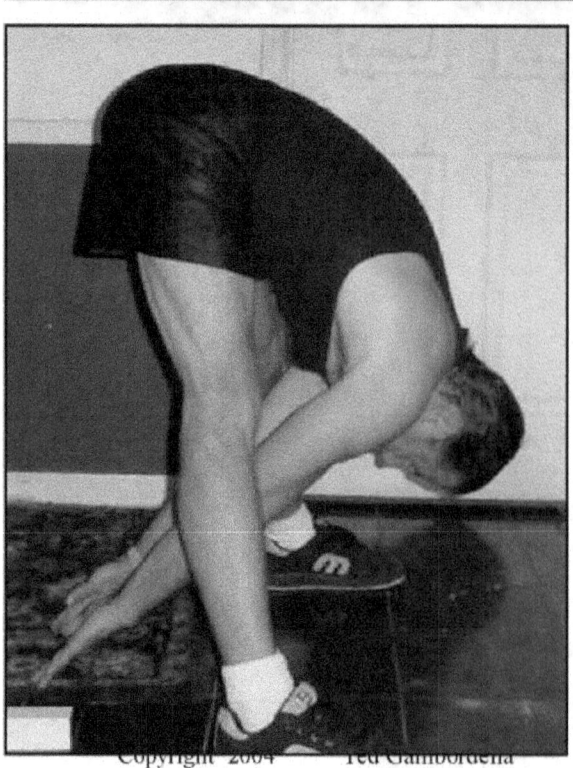

Here we lean over and do a step reach back, go further back with each step.

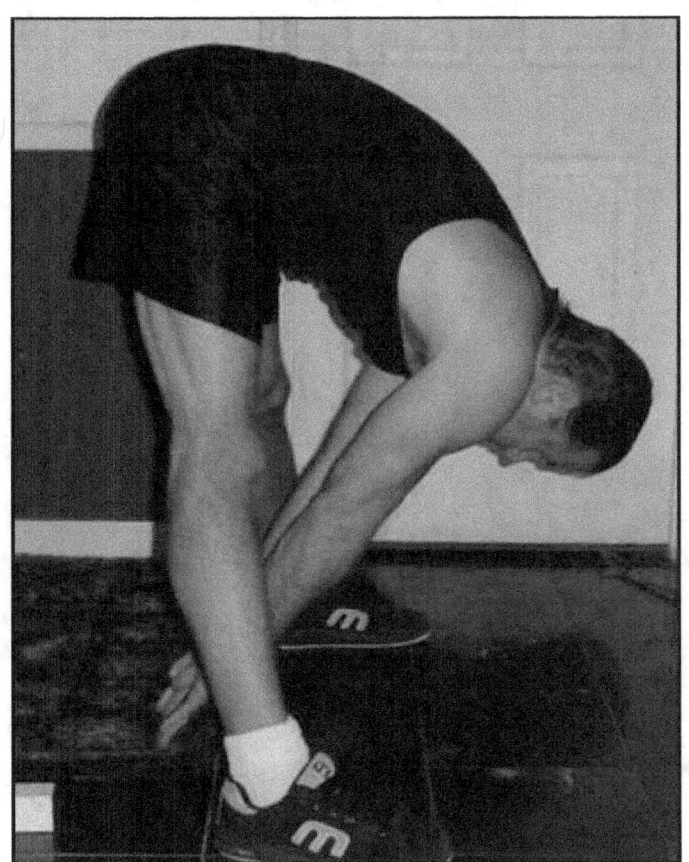

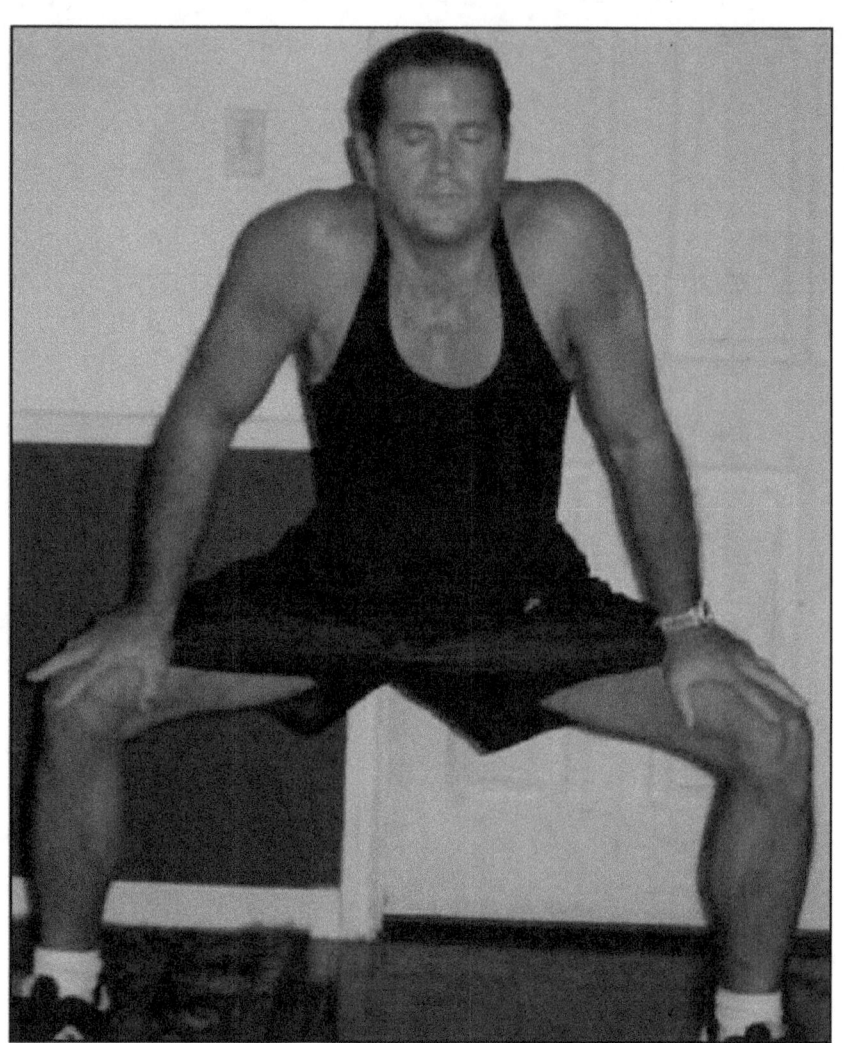

Squat down and place the arms on top of the knees. Let the body settle here..

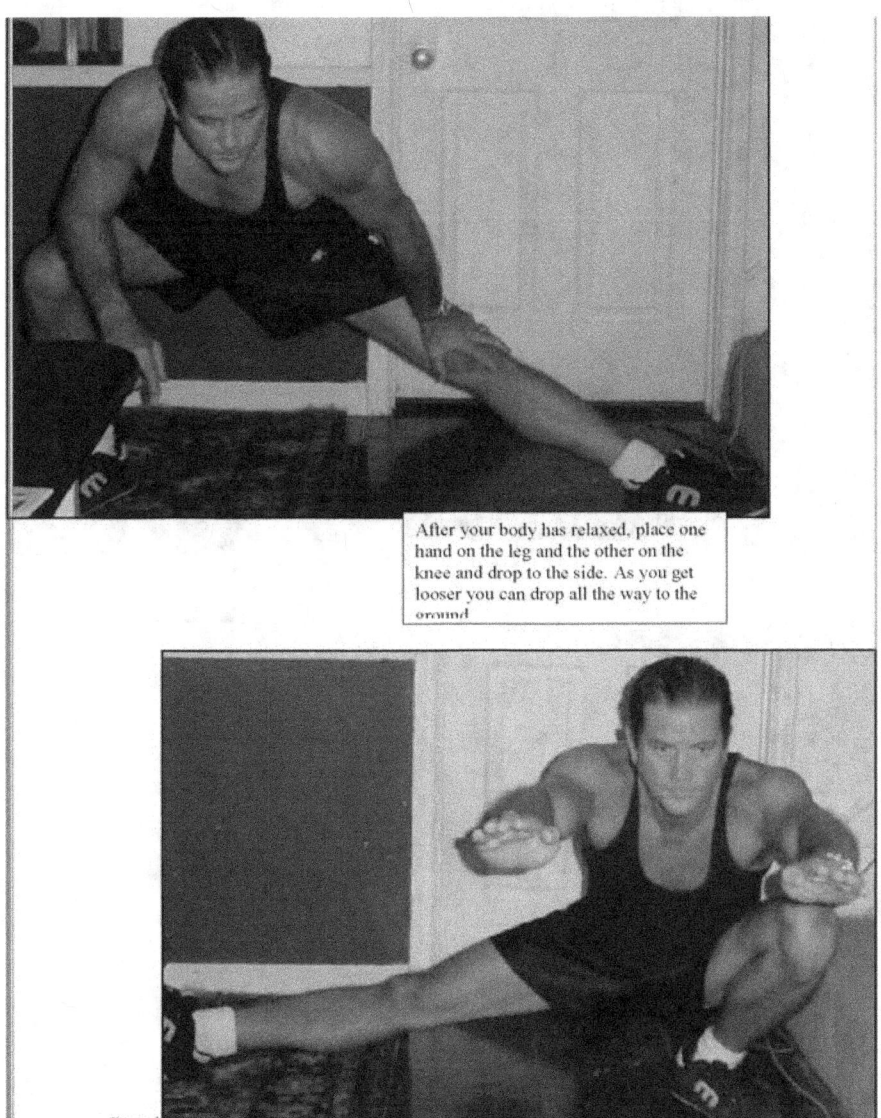

After your body has relaxed, place one hand on the leg and the other on the knee and drop to the side. As you get looser you can drop all the way to the ground.

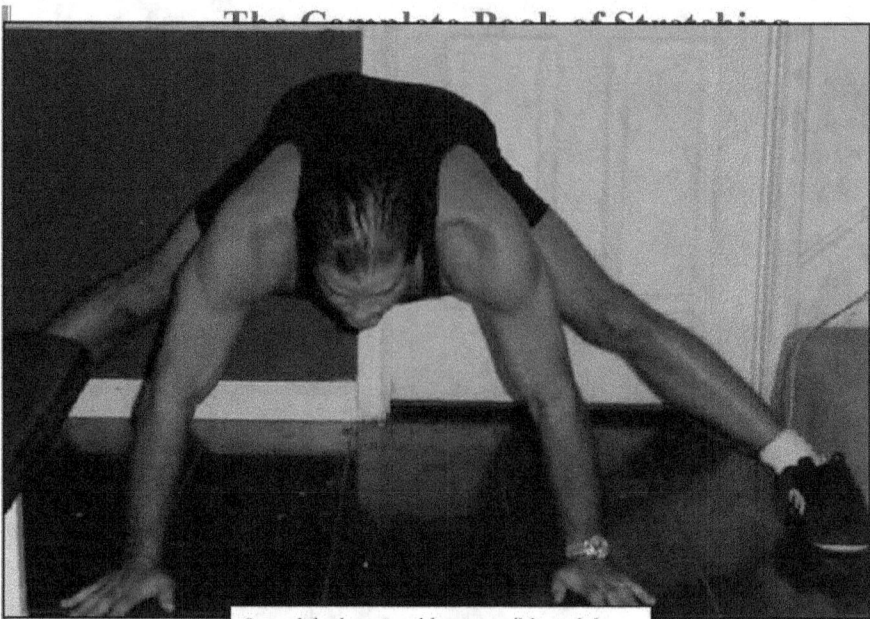

Spread the legs as wide as possible and then
put the hands on the ground. Try to relax and
touch the head to the ground.

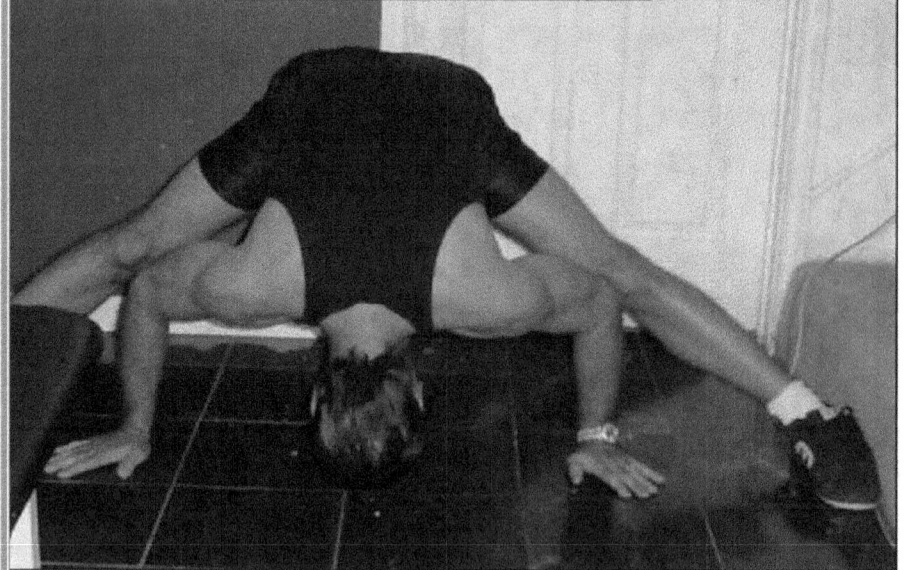

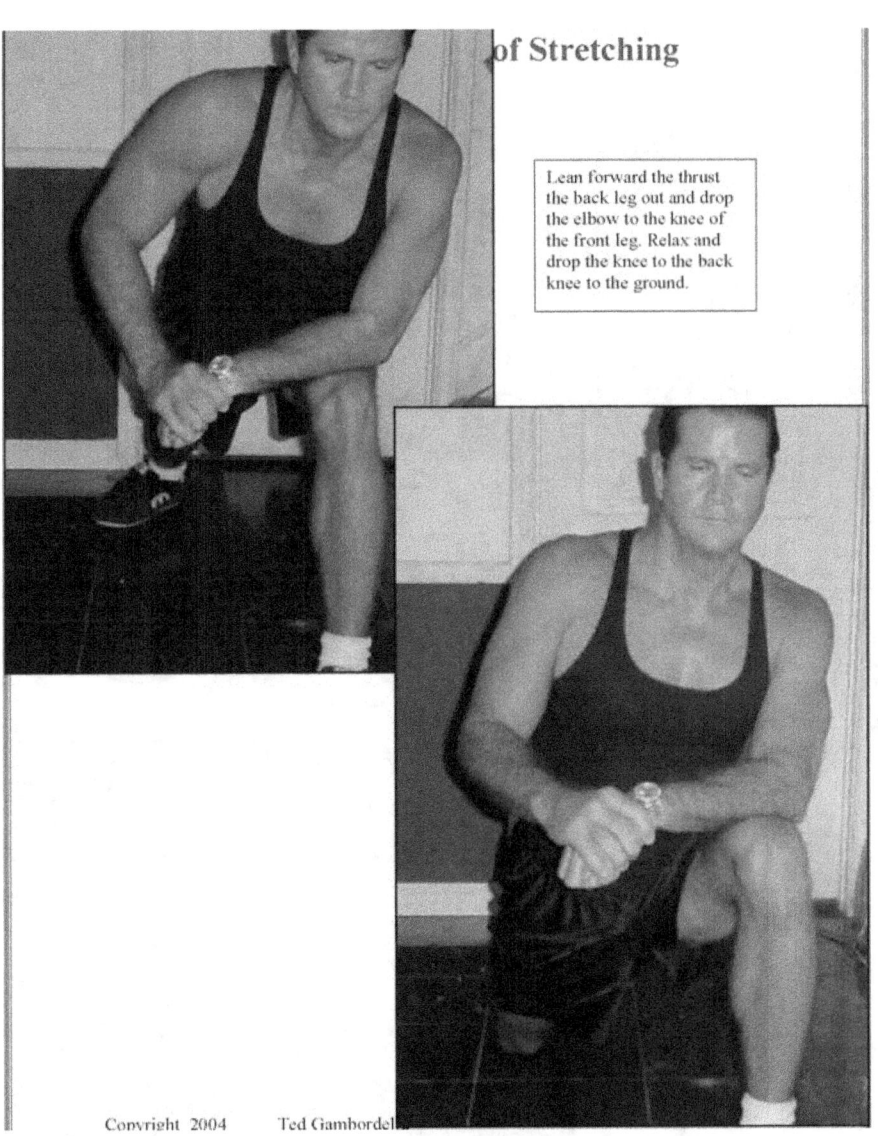

Lean forward the thrust
the back leg out and drop
the elbow to the knee of
the front leg. Relax and
drop the knee to the back
knee to the ground.

Spread the leg as wide as possible forward and backwards, try to drop the hips to the ground on both sides.

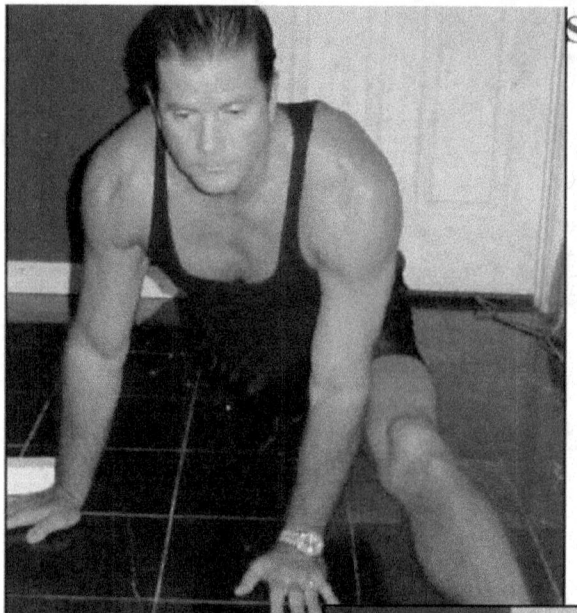

Stretching

Spread the leg as wide as possible forward and backwards, try to drop the hips to the ground on both sides.

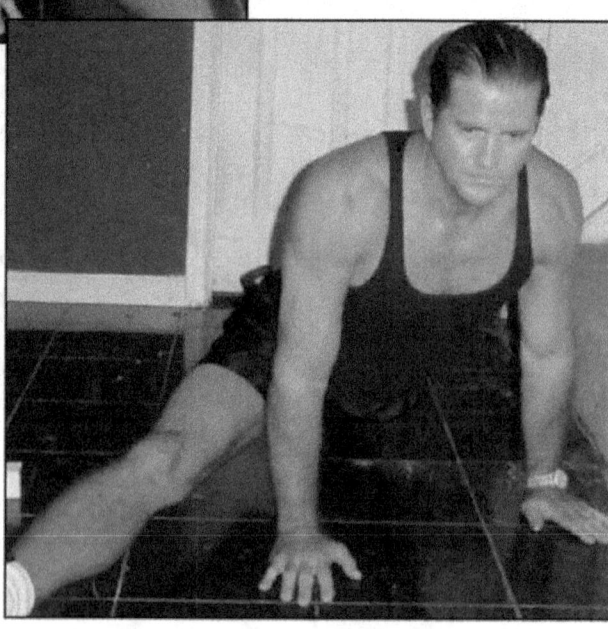

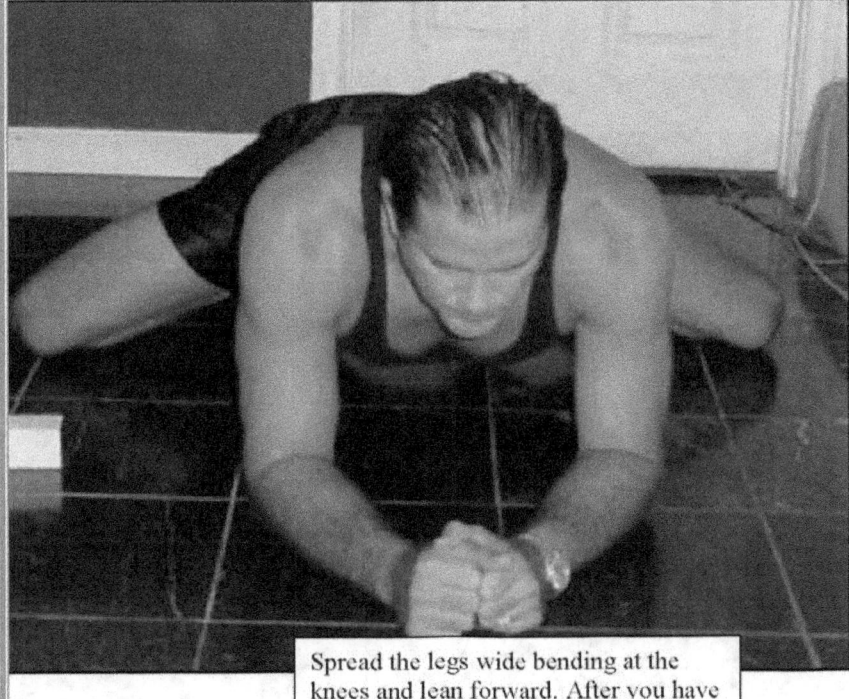

Spread the legs wide bending at the knees and lean forward. After you have relaxed, try to drop the hips to the ground.

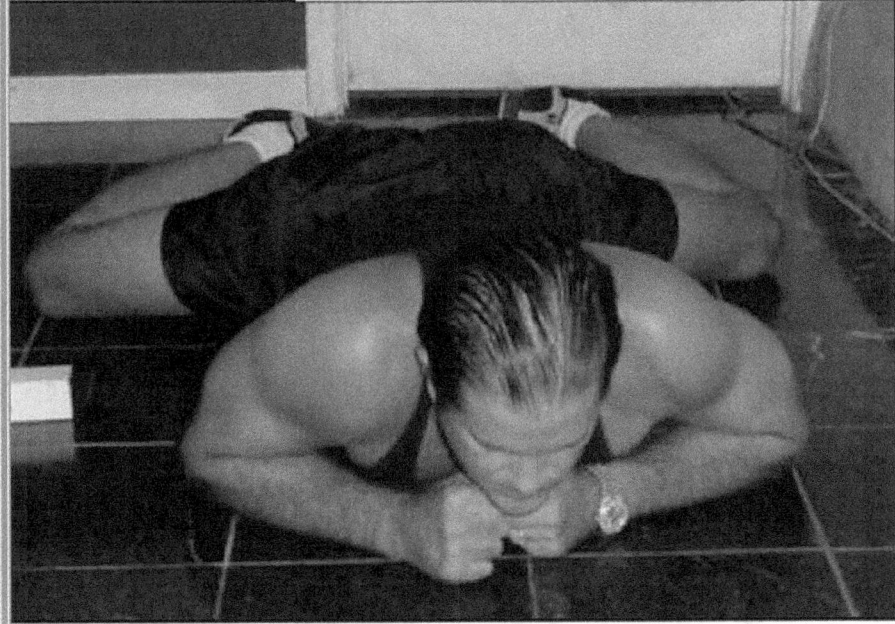

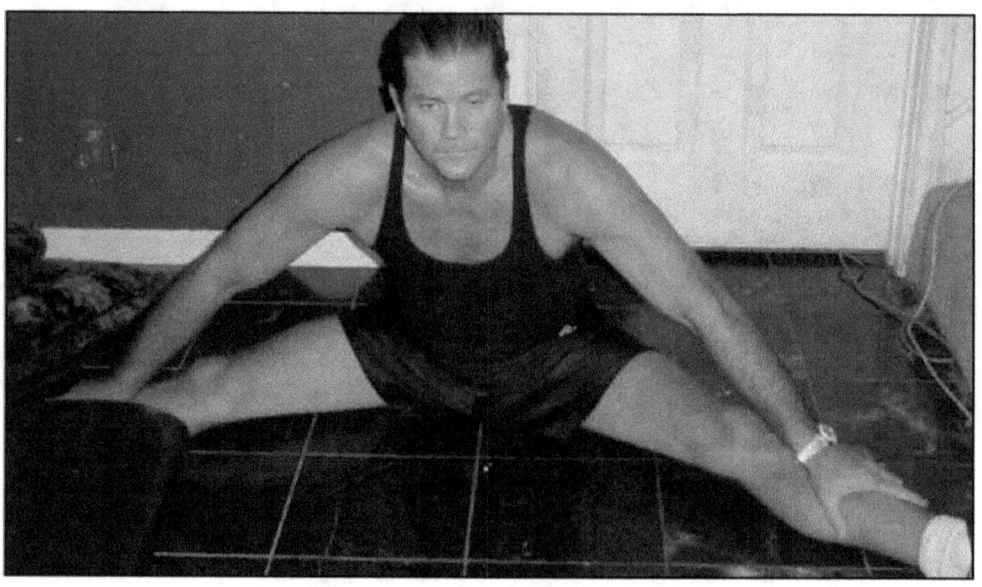

Sit on the floor and spread the legs as wide as possible. Lean slowly forward to loosen up.

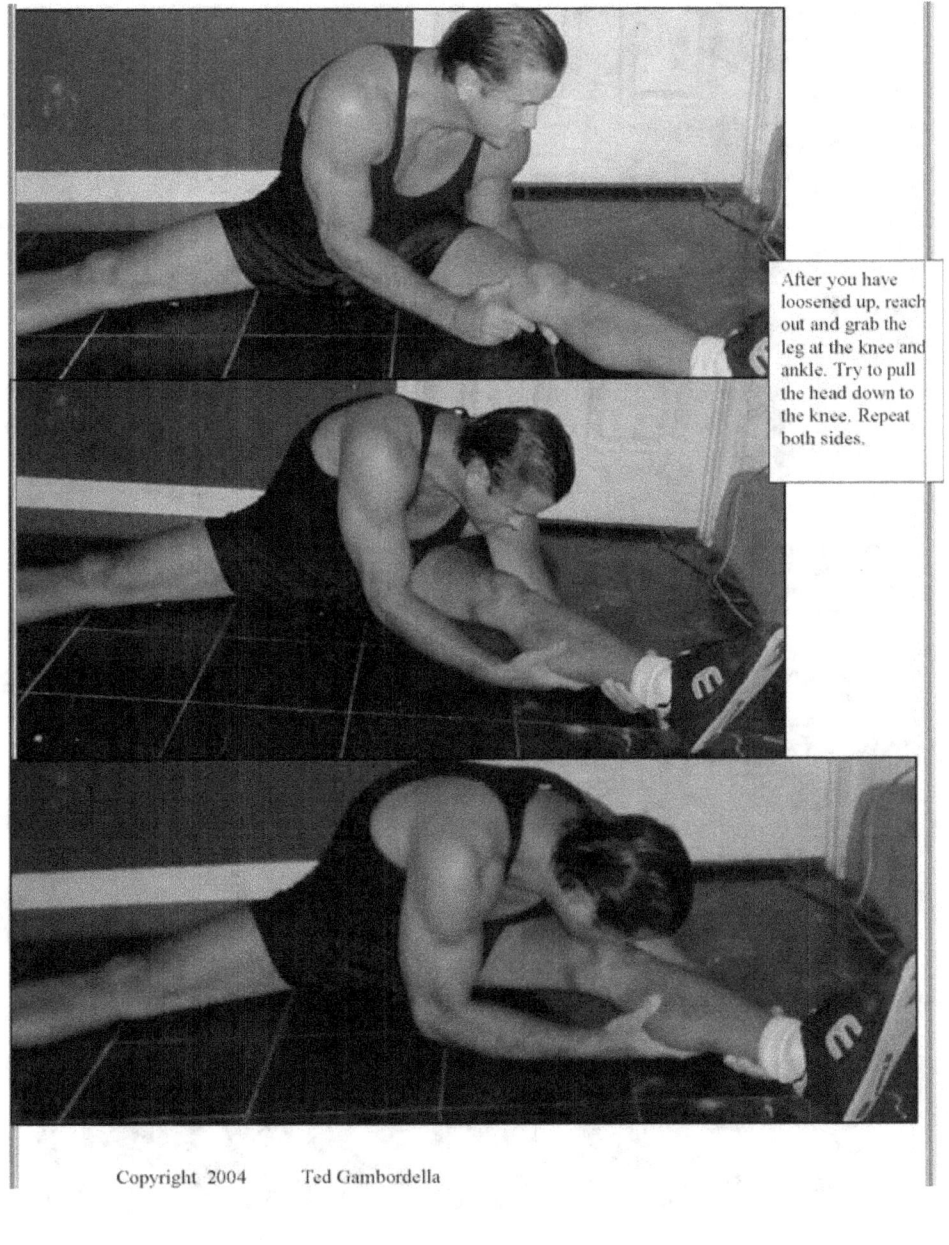

After you have loosened up, reach out and grab the leg at the knee and ankle. Try to pull the head down to the knee. Repeat both sides.

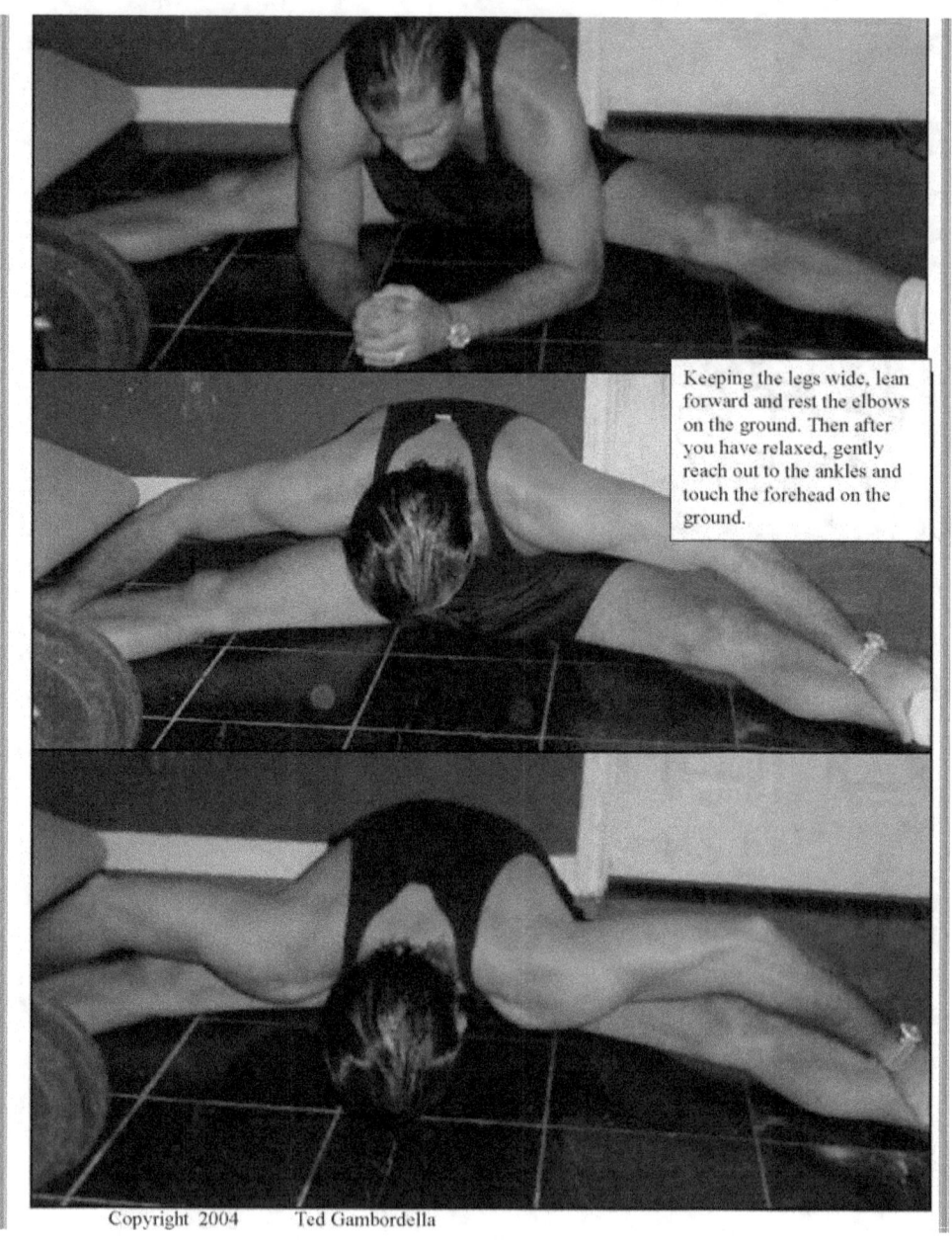

Keeping the legs wide, lean forward and rest the elbows on the ground. Then after you have relaxed, gently reach out to the ankles and touch the forehead on the ground.

Copyright 2004   Ted Gambordella

Sitting on the ground. Put the balls of your feet together and while holding the ankles gently rock the legs trying to get them to the ground. You can help by pushing down on the knees.

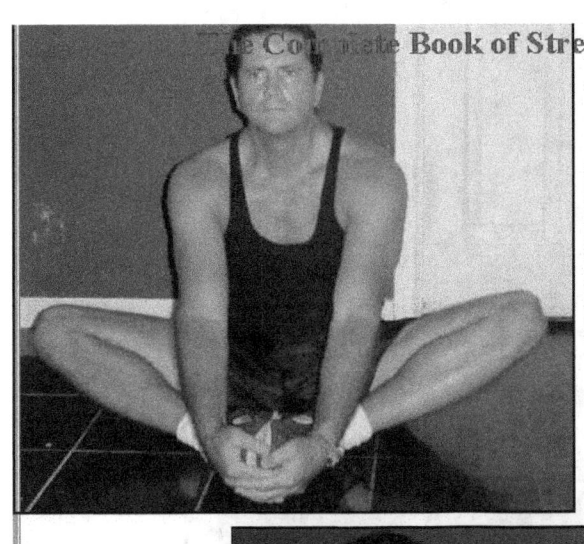

Sitting on the ground. Put the balls of your feet together and while holding the ankles gently rock the legs trying to get them to the ground. You can help by pushing down on the knees.

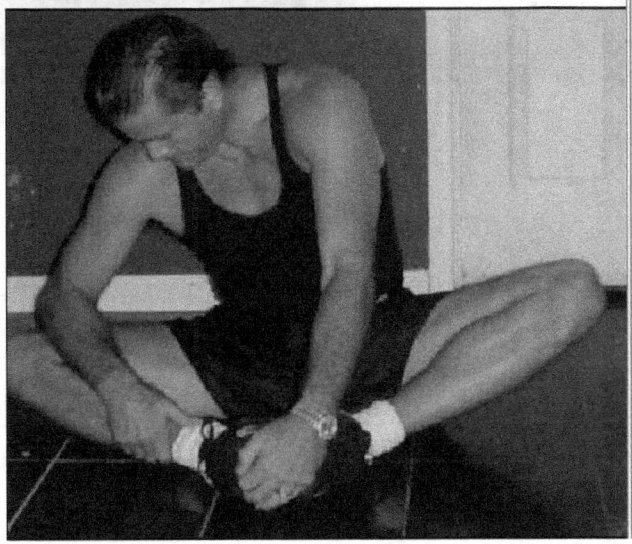

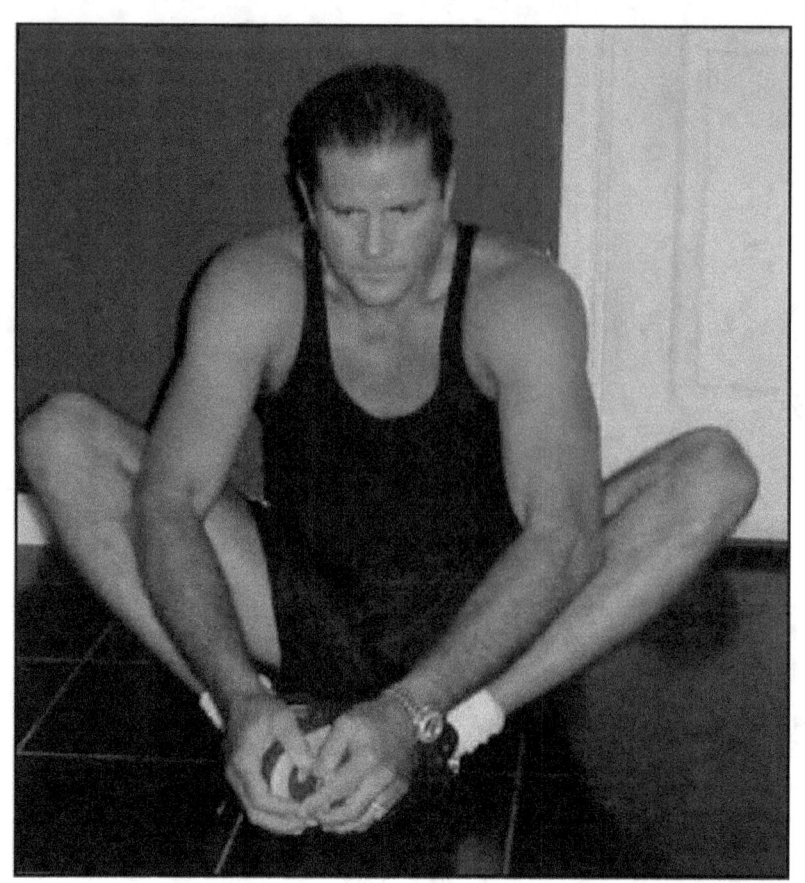

After you have relaxed, you can hold onto the ankles and try to touch the head to

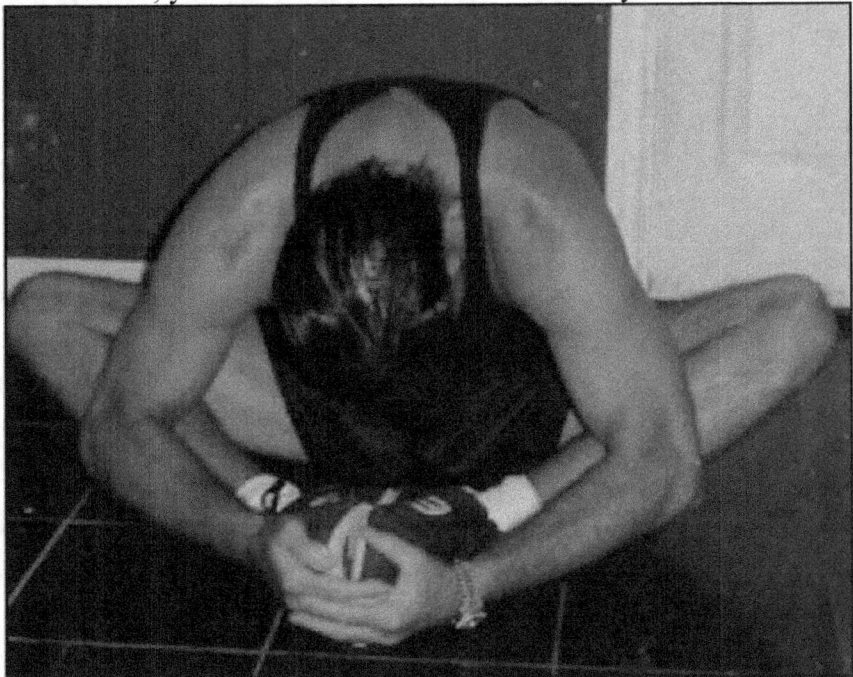

the ankles.

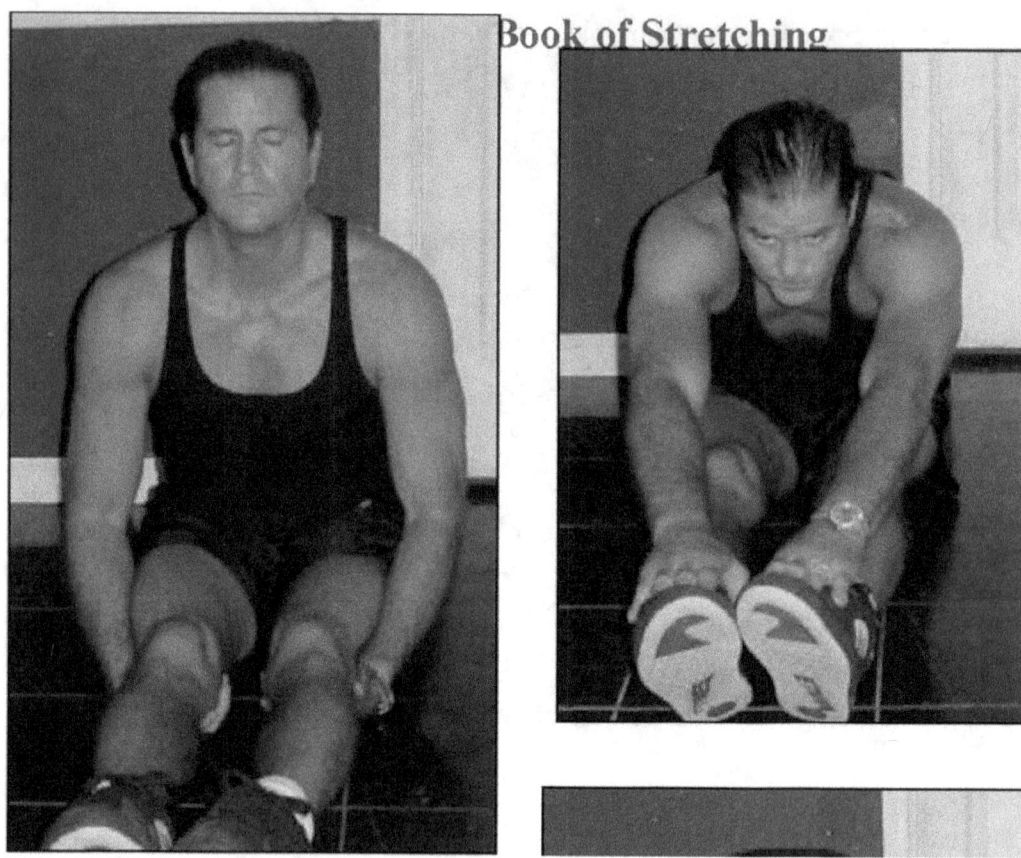

Sit with both legs directly out to the front of the body and then reach out to try to touch the toes. As you loosen up reach down and touch the head to the knees.

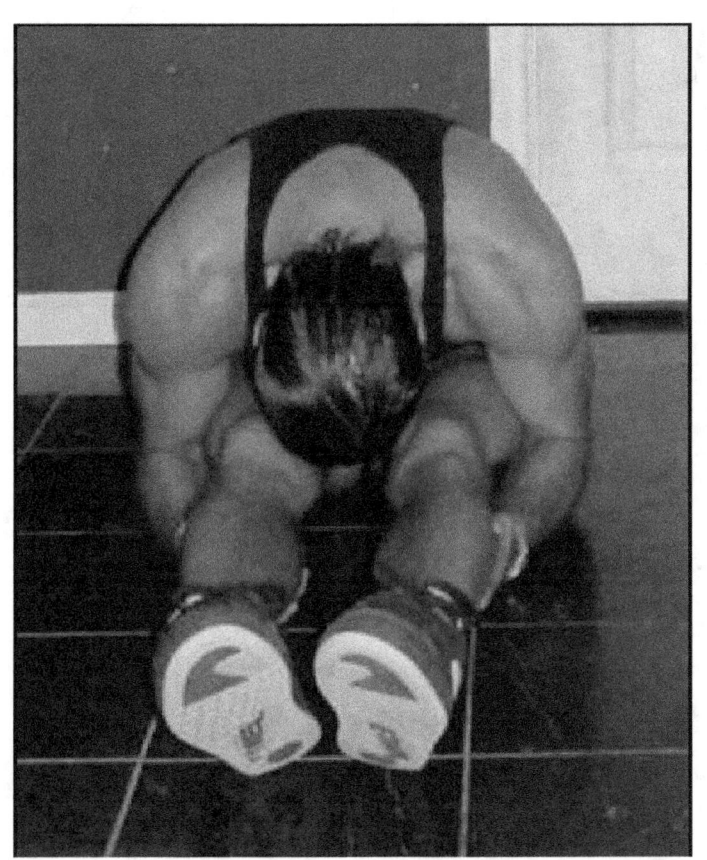

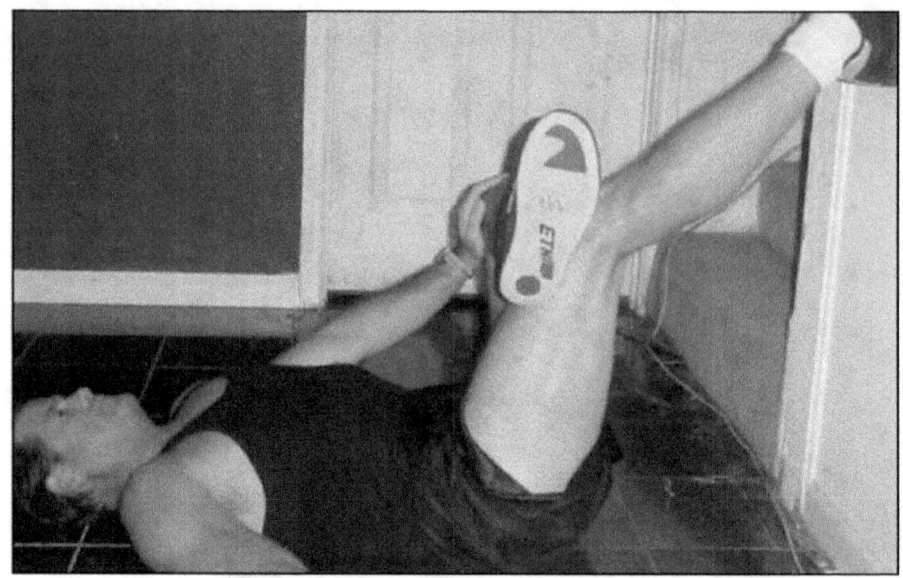

Put one leg against the wall and cross the leg over the knee to loosen the hips.

Lying on the back, reach down and grab the leg and pull it as high as you can towards your head.

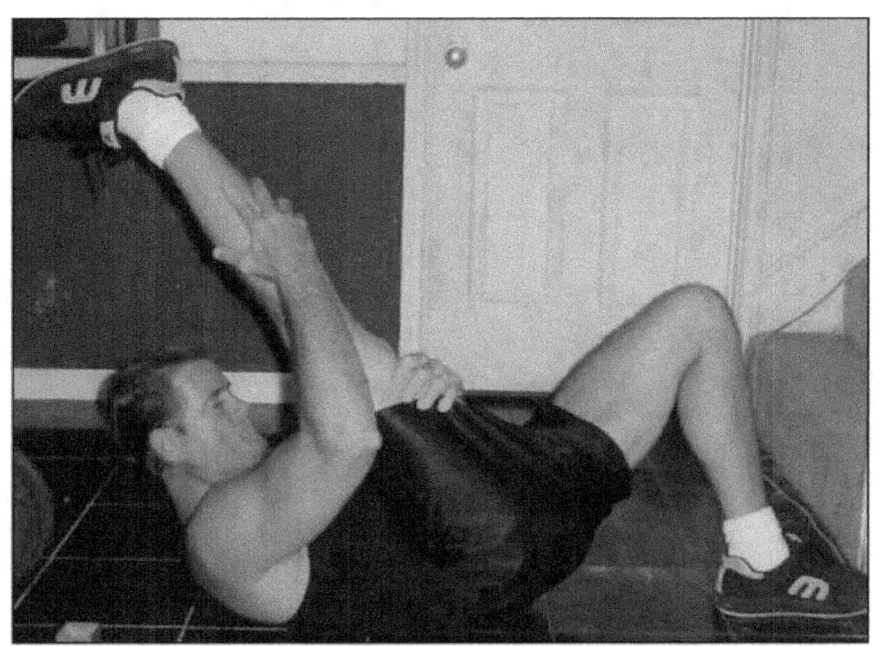

Reach down and grab the knee and pull it into the chest.

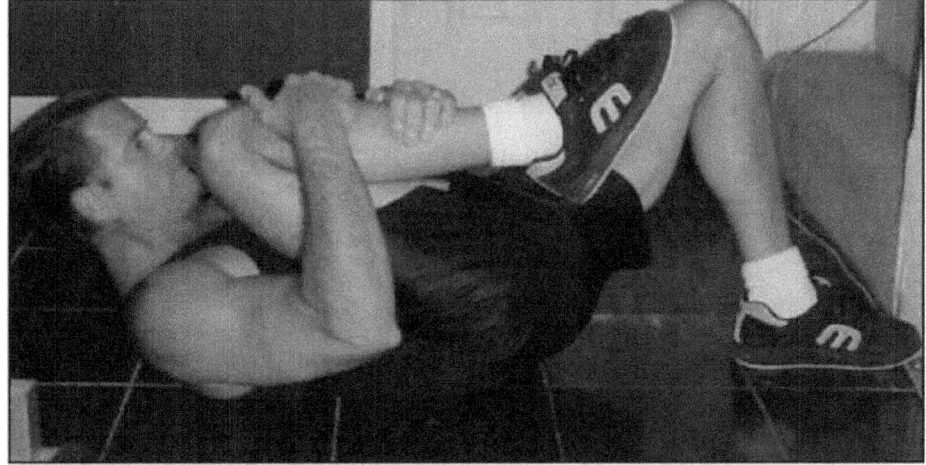

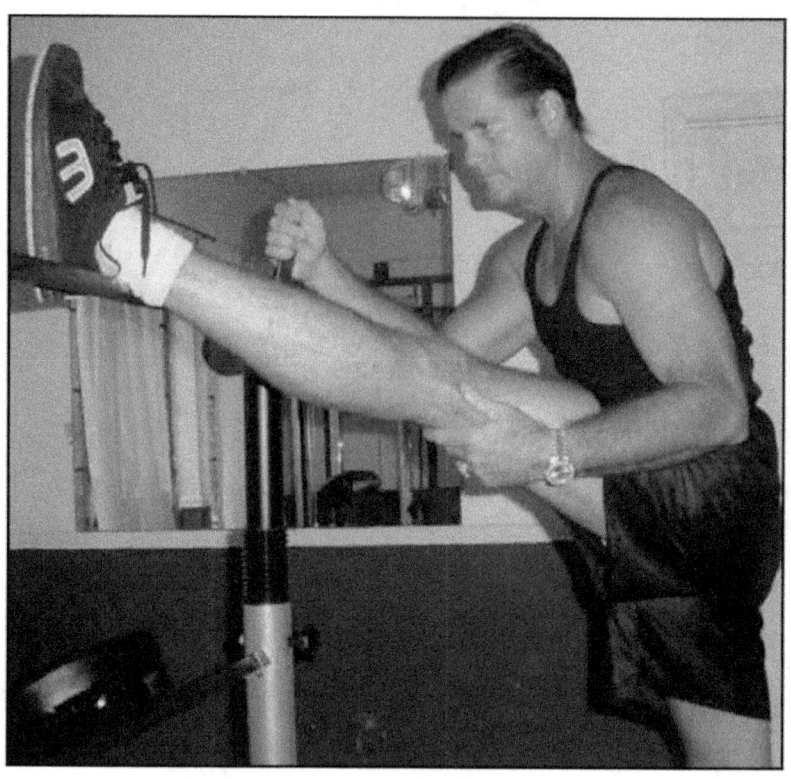

Place the leg on a bar or table and keep the knee locked out. Then lean over and touch the head to the knee.

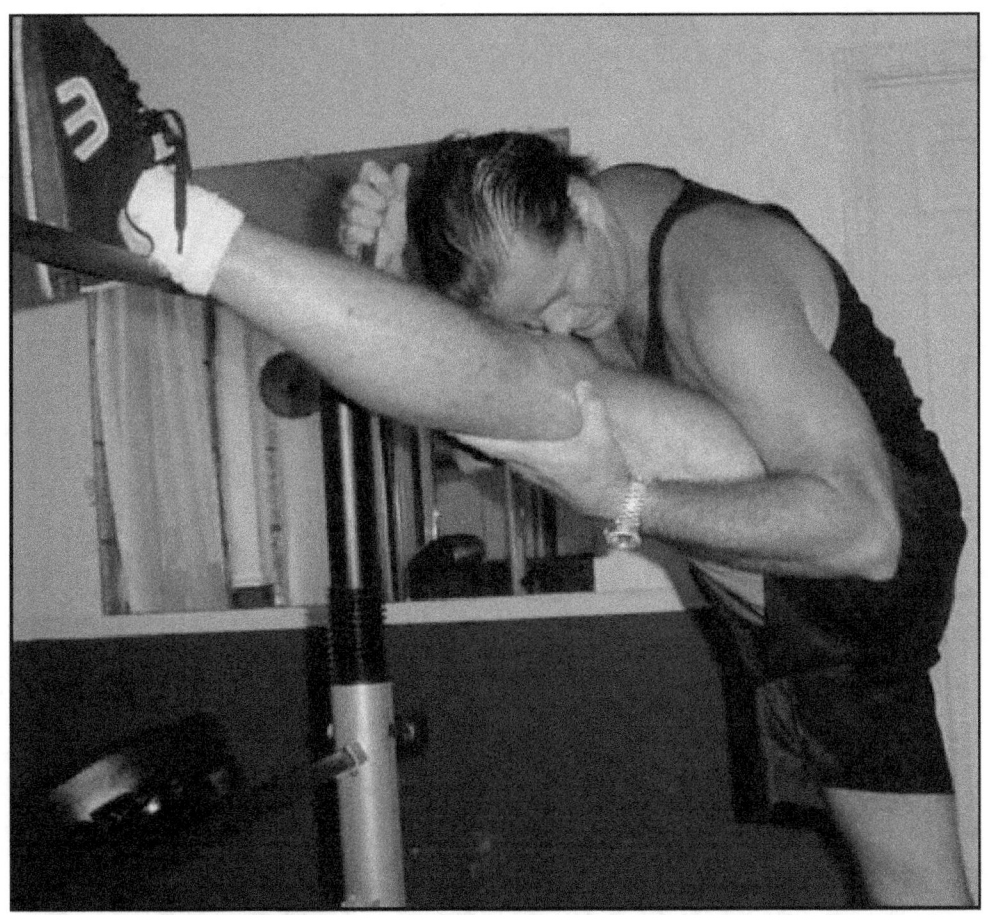

Sit in chair. Move heel of involved leg under chair. Place other leg in front and push back. Hold stretch, relax, and repeat.

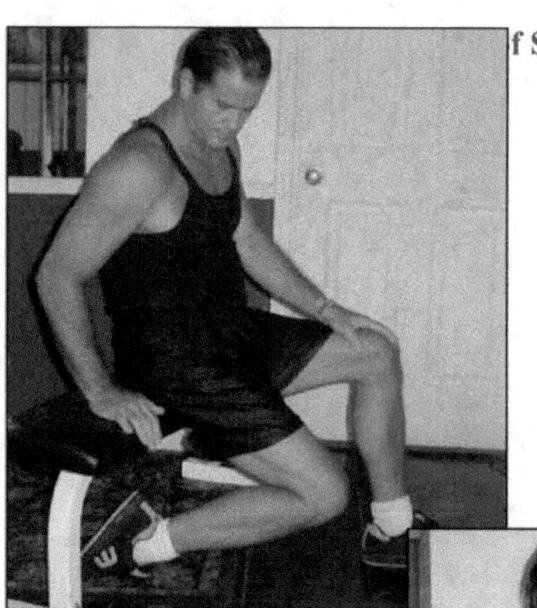

Sit in chair.
Move heel of involved leg under chair.
Place other leg in front and push back.
Hold stretch, relax, and repeat.

Stretch the hamstrings by
leaning into the wall and
dropping the kneed to the
ground.

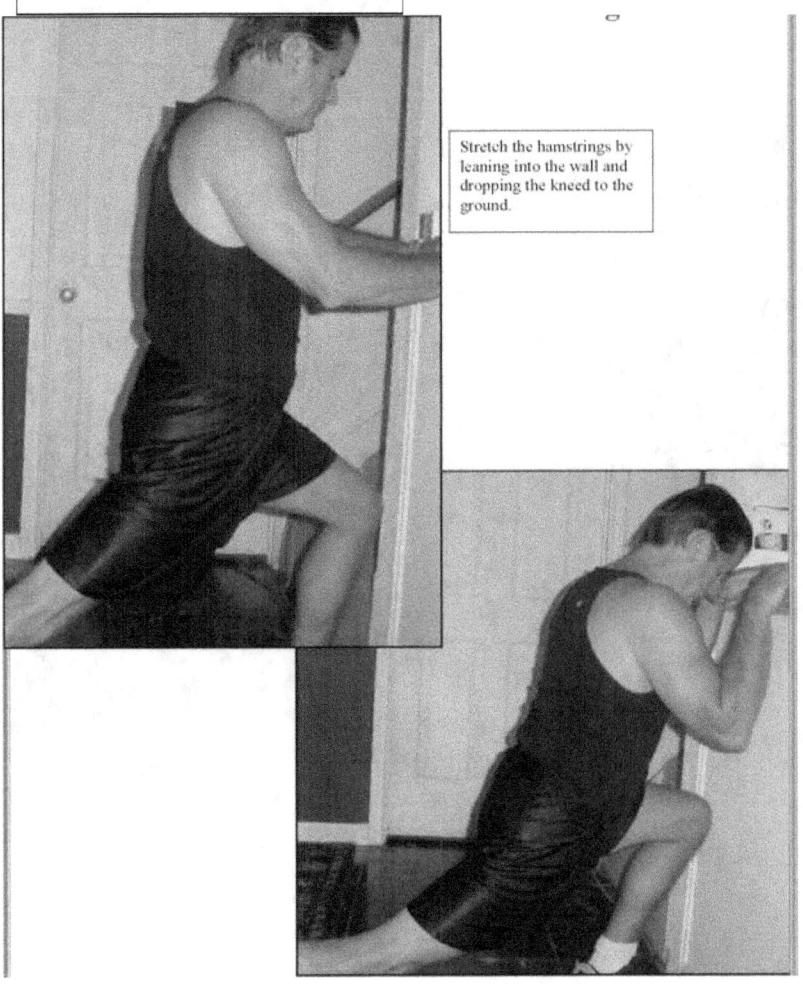

Stretch the hamstrings by
leaning into the wall and
dropping the kneed to the
ground.

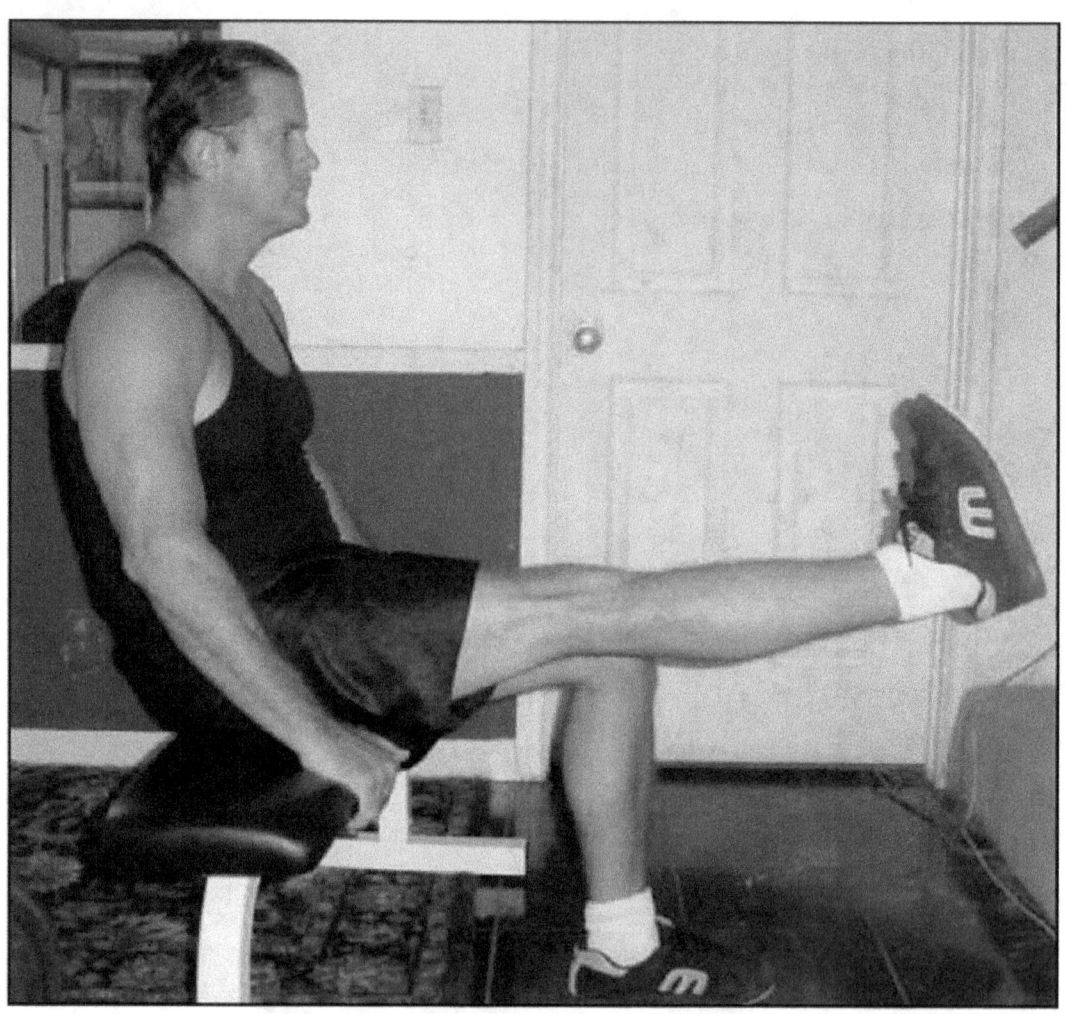

Stretch the calf by holding the leg out straight and pulling back with the ankle.

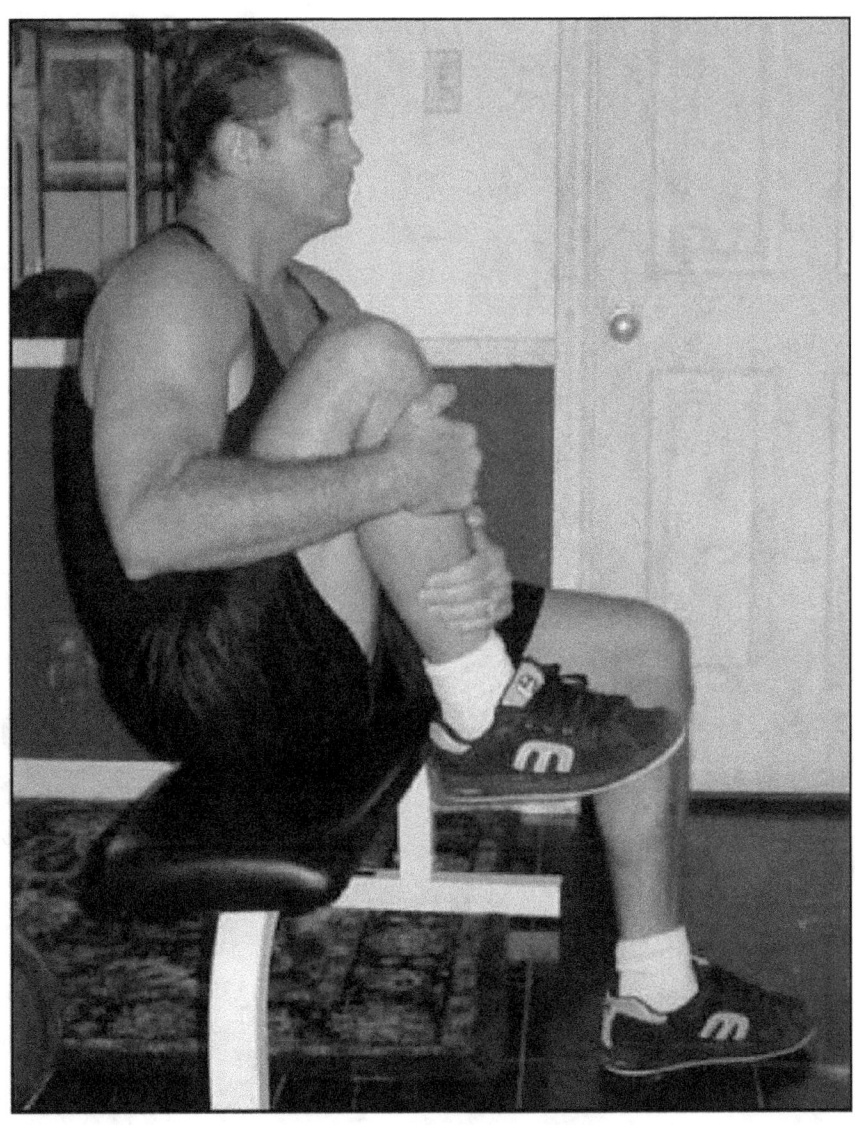

Reach down and grab the knee and pull it to the chest.

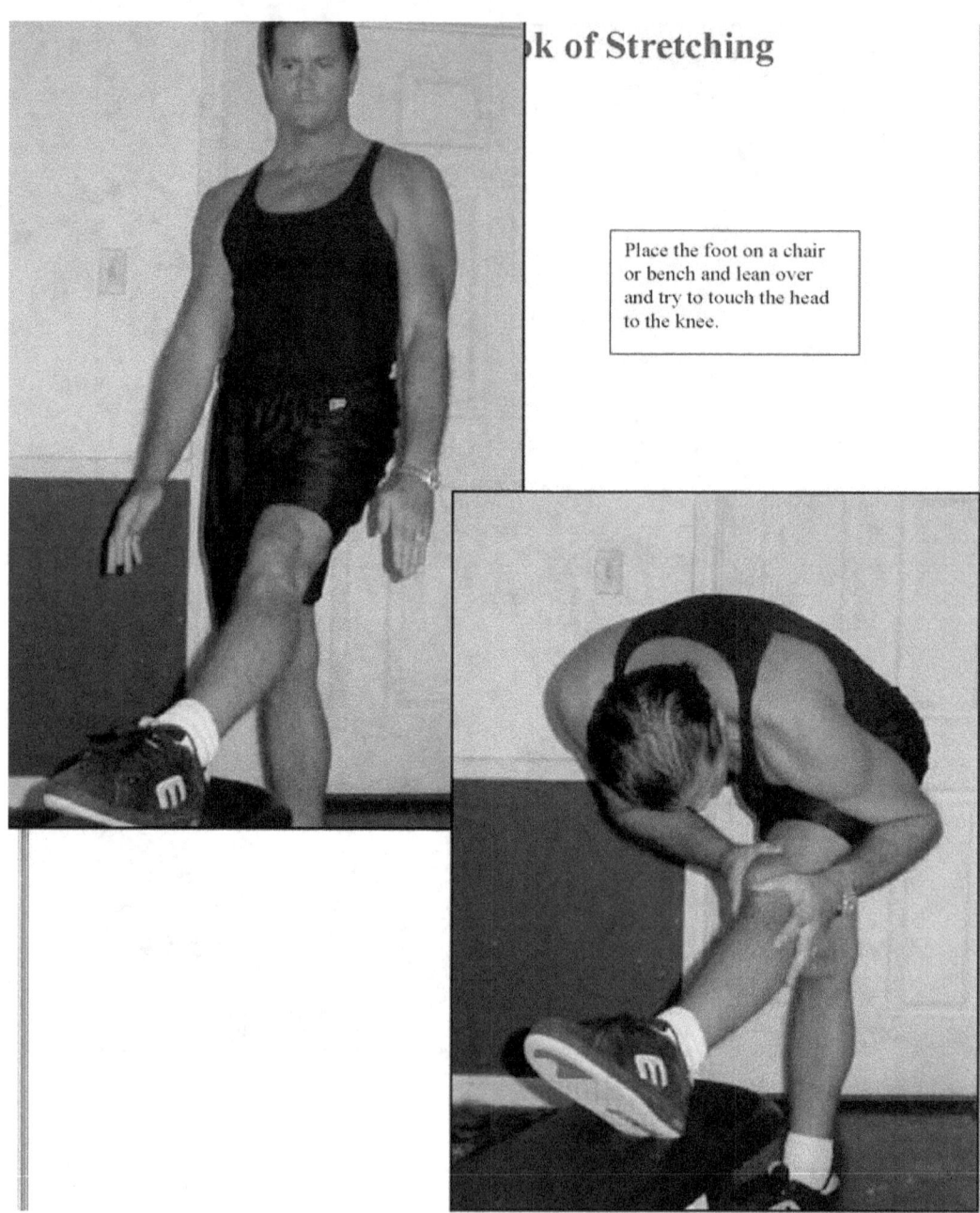

Place the foot on a chair or bench and lean over and try to touch the head to the knee.

Lie on the back with the legs on the wall, then let the legs separate and spread as wide as possible

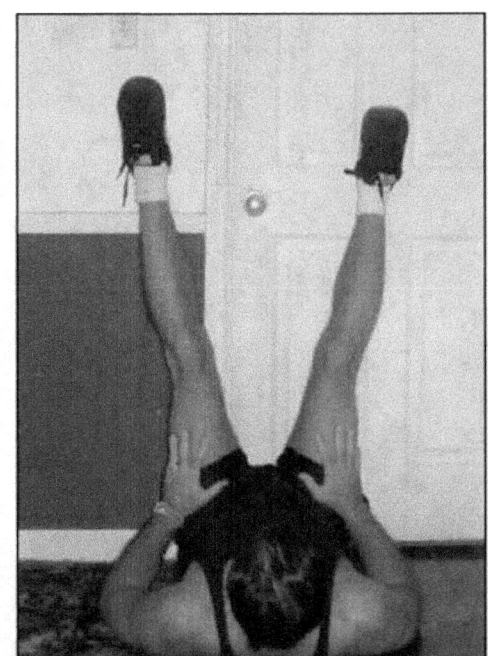

Lie on the back with the
legs on the wall, then let
the legs separate and
spread as wide as
possible.

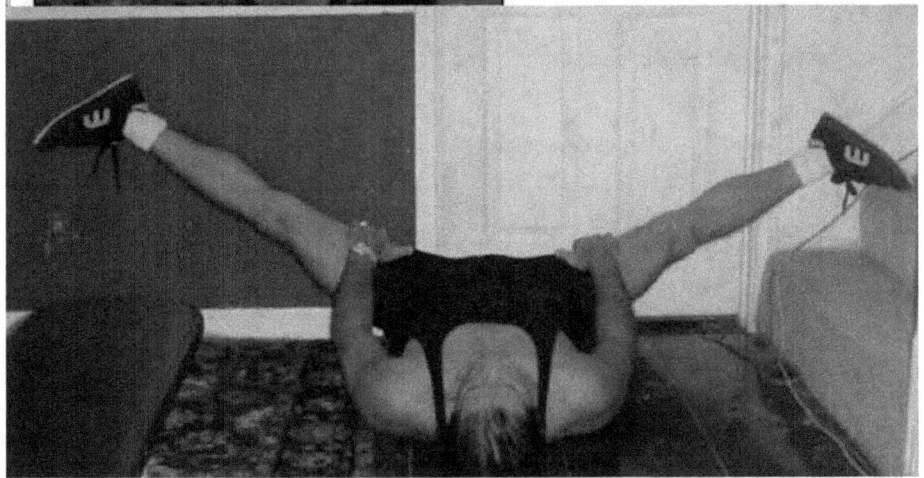

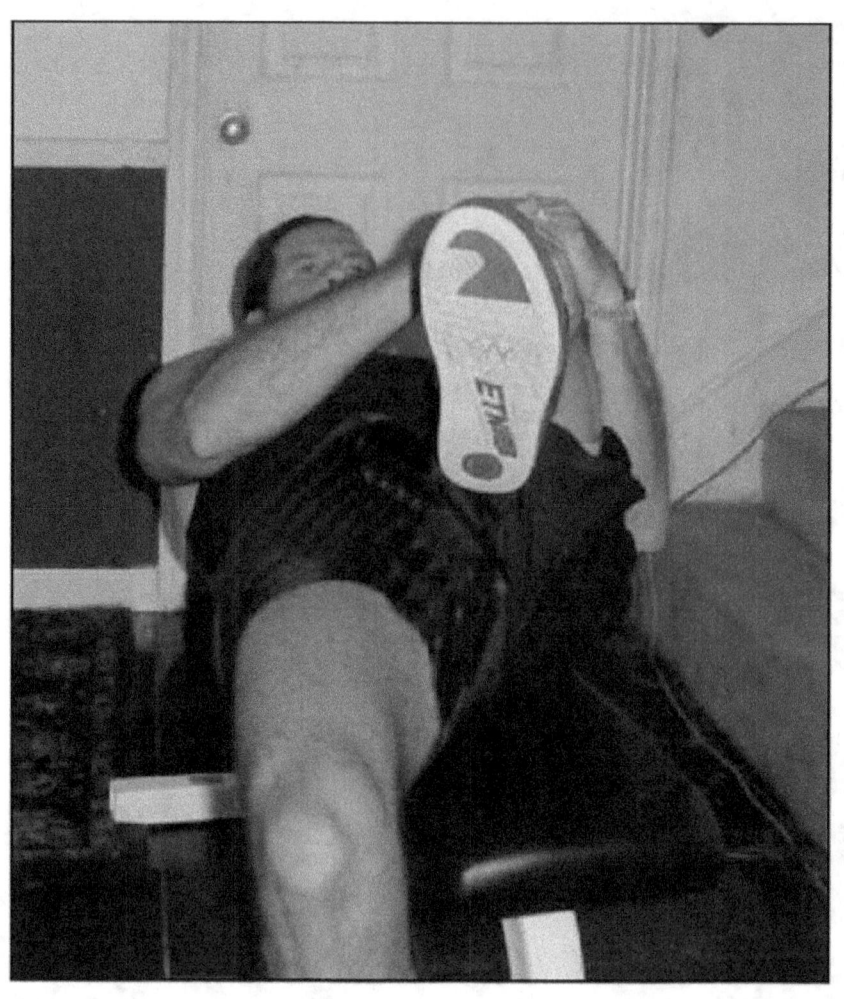

Lie on your back on the bench and reach down and pull the knee up to the chest.

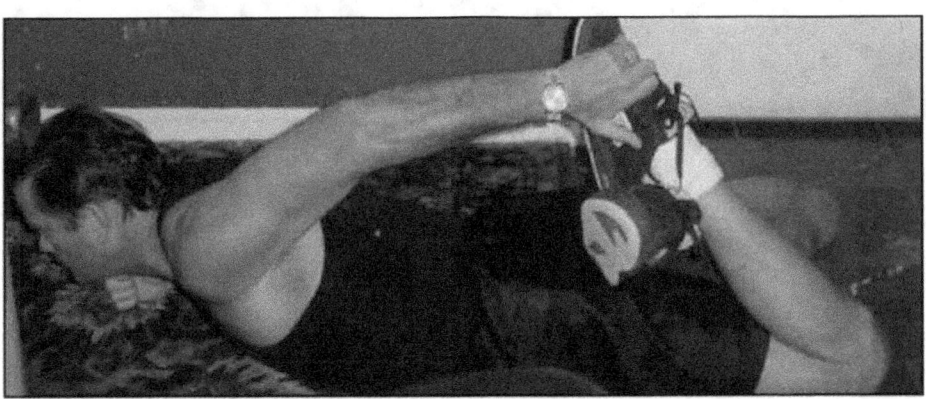

Lie on your stomach and cross the legs, then reach up and grab the ankle of one leg and pull.

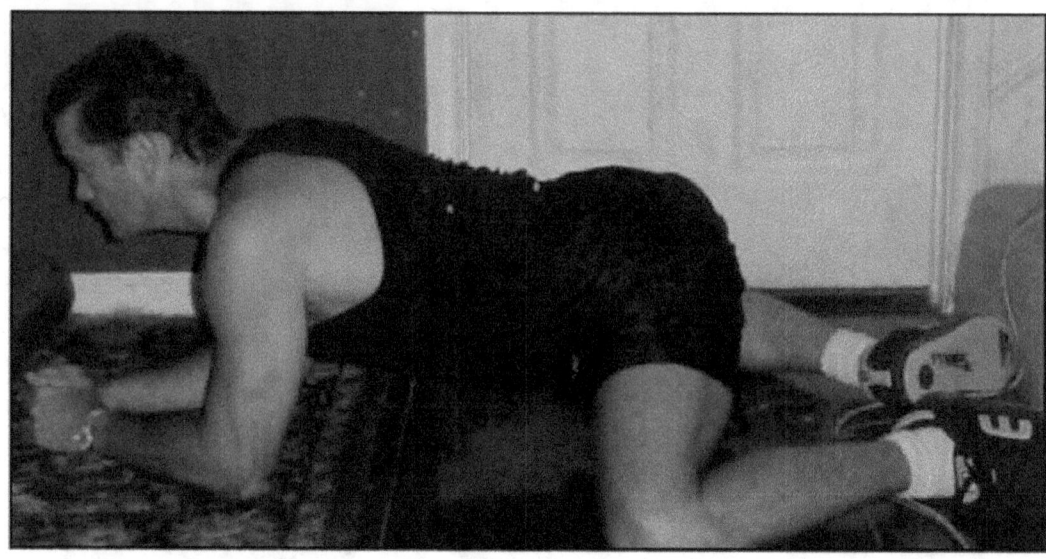

Here we lie on the floor on our knees and elbows. Relax, breath, and try to move the hips to the ground.

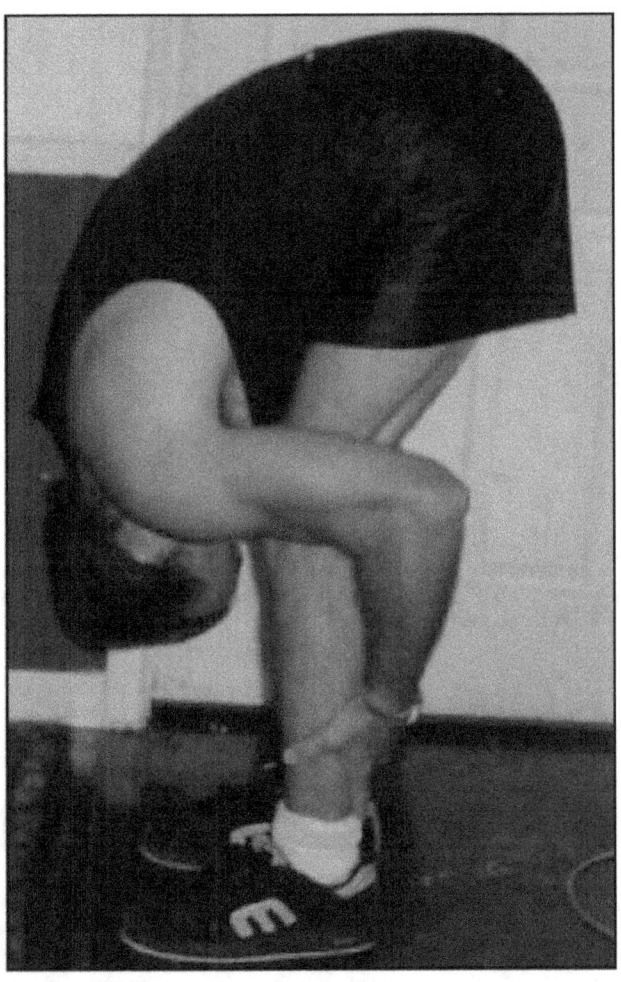

This stretch is difficult but can be done after much practice and relaxation. Simply bend over and grab the knees, touching the head.

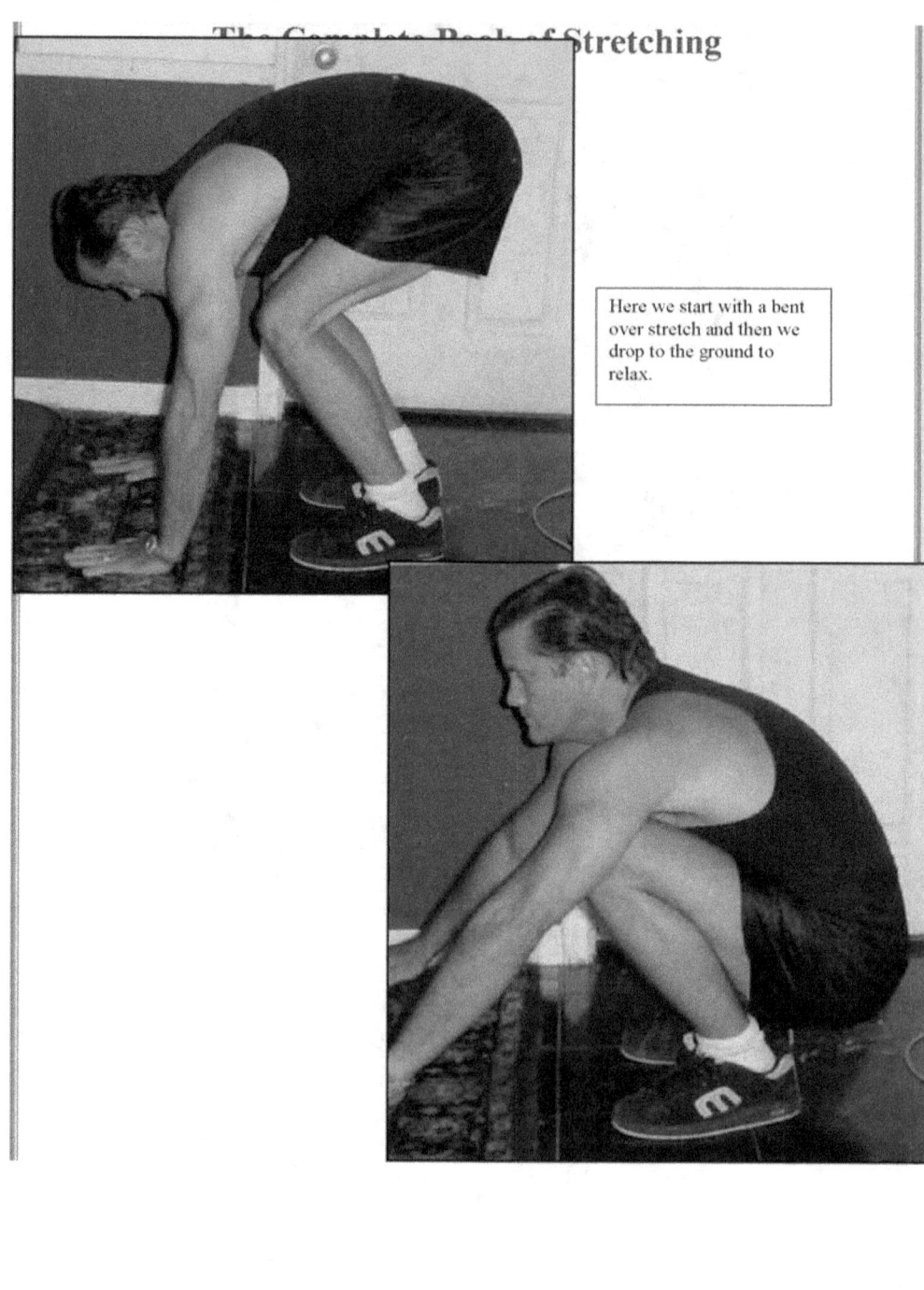

Here we start with a bent over stretch and then we drop to the ground to relax.

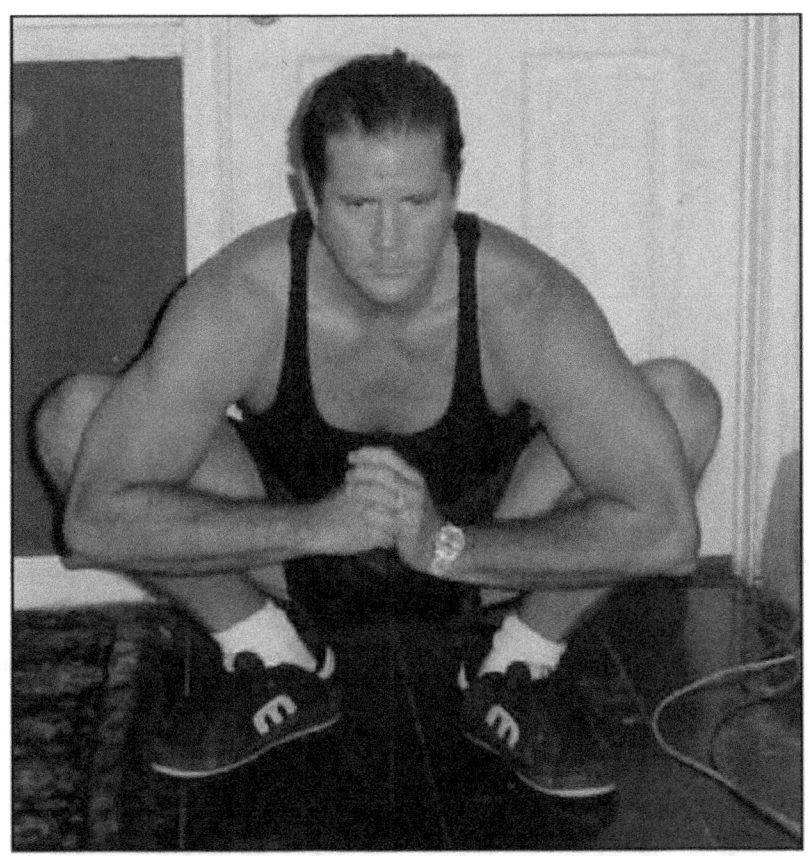

Sit down on the heels and drop the buttock to the floor then push out on the knees with the elbows.

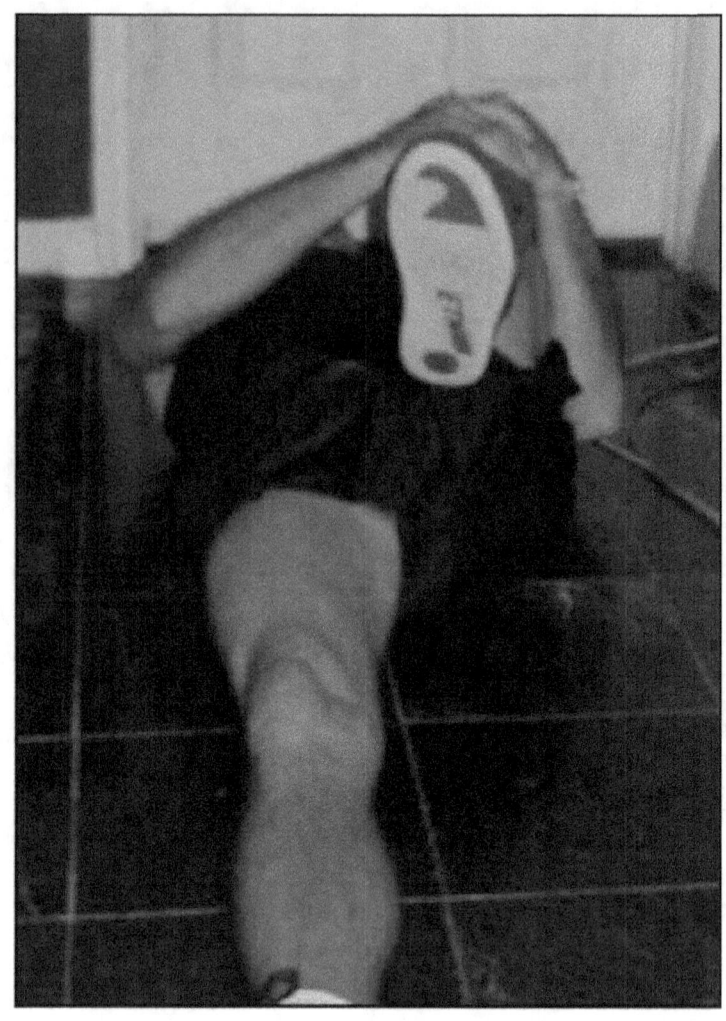

Lie on the back and reach down and pull up the leg to the chest, alternating sides.

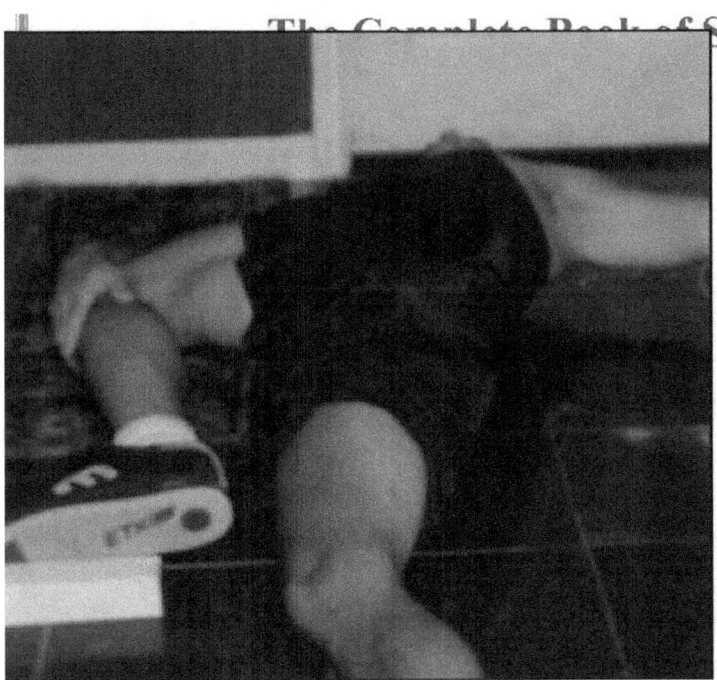

Continue
holding t
dropping
alternati

Continue this stretch by holding the knee and dropping it to the floor on

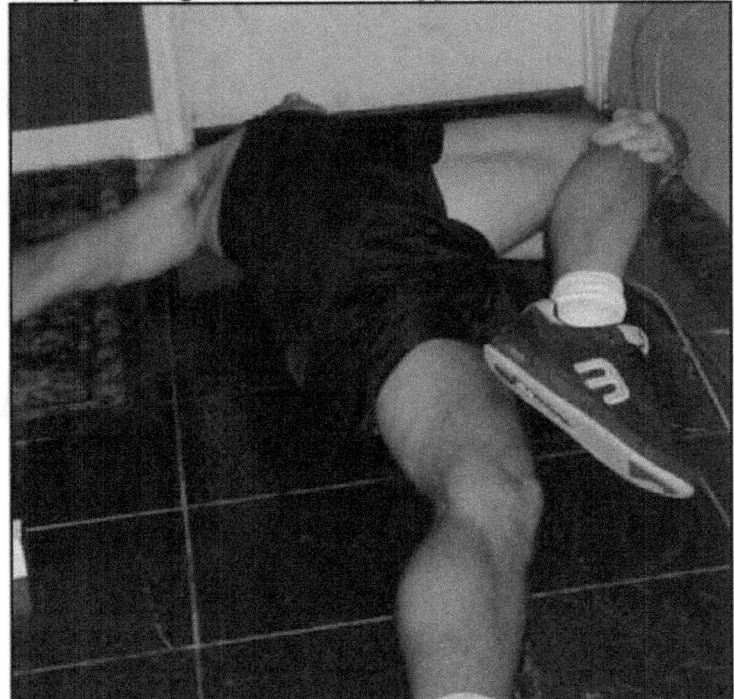

alternating sides.

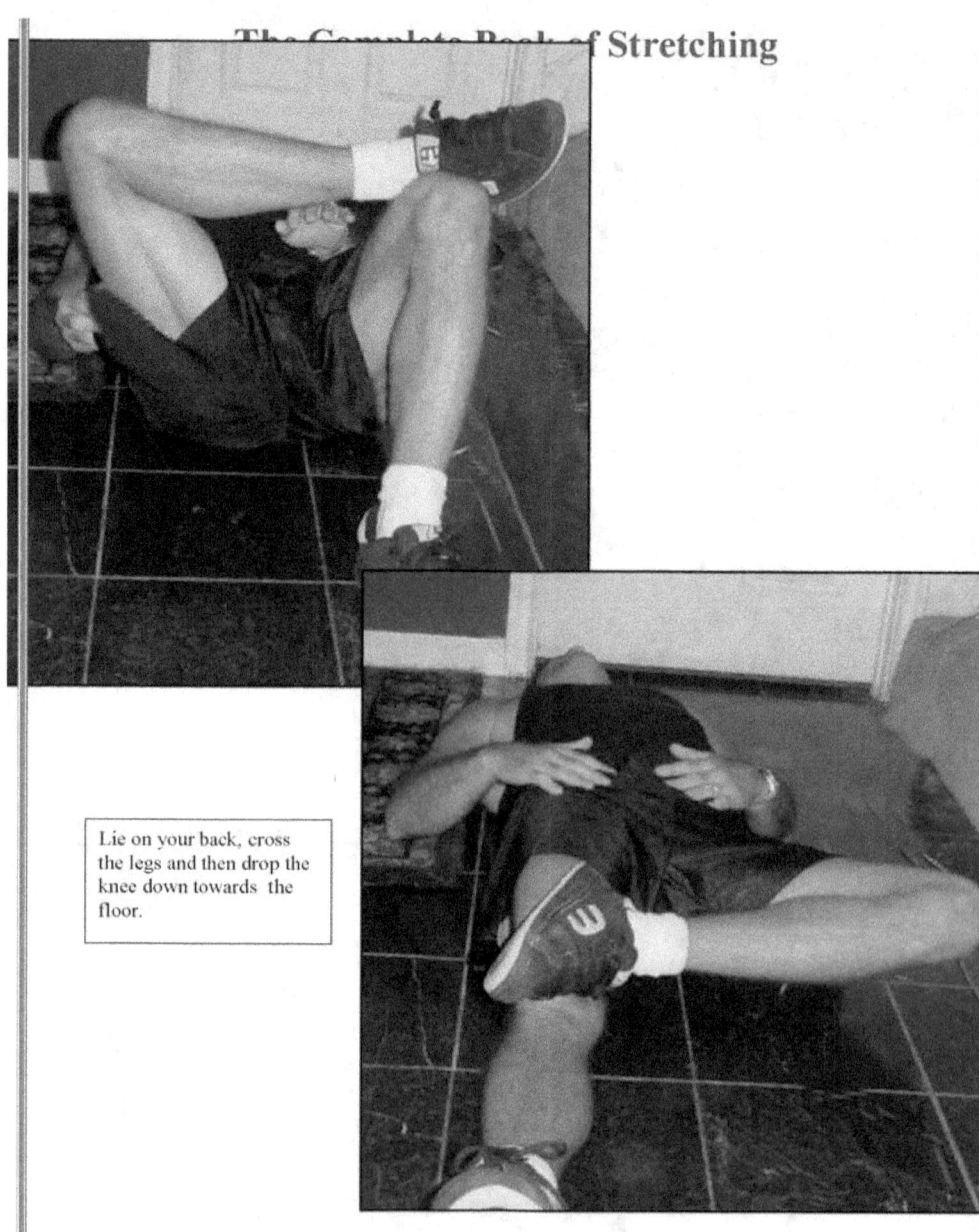

Lie on your back, cross the legs and then drop the knee down towards the floor.

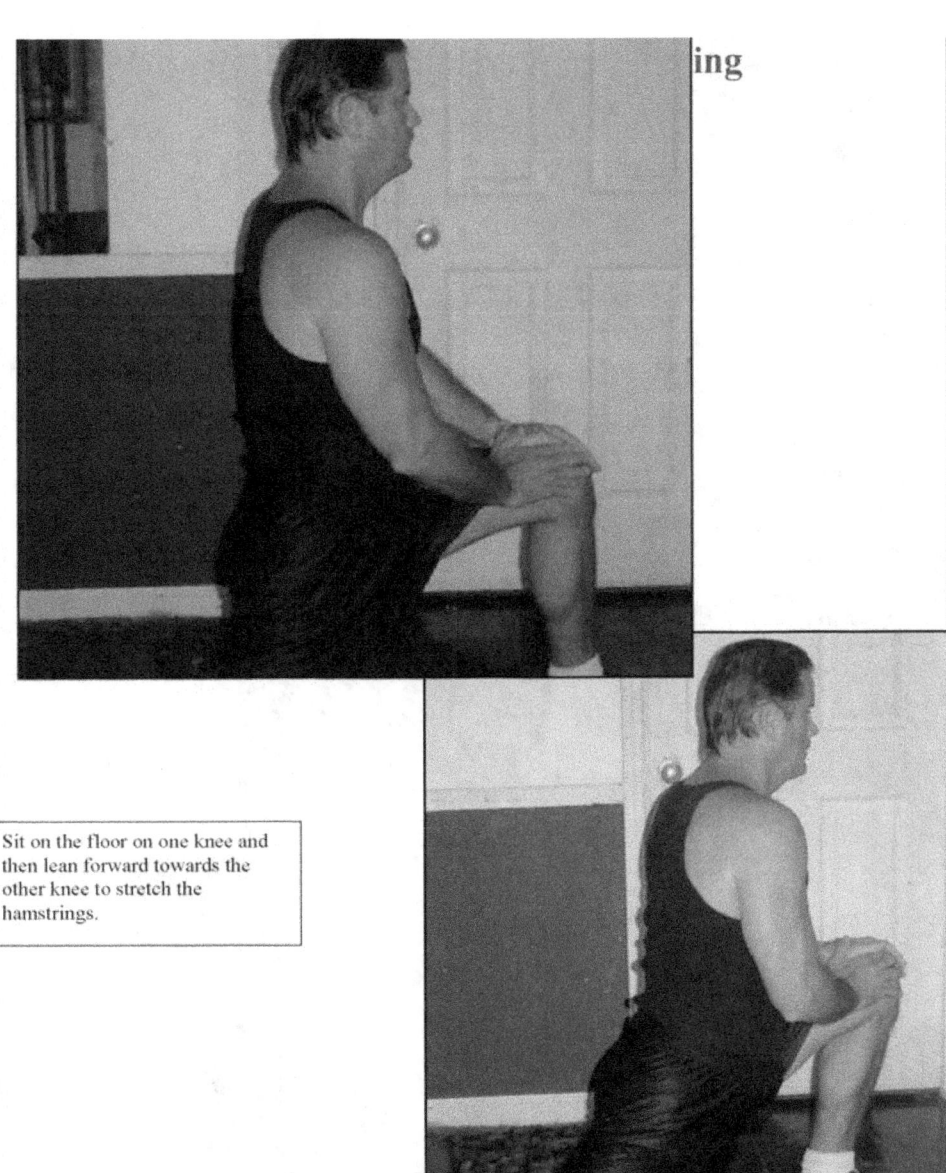

Sit on the floor on one knee and
then lean forward towards the
other knee to stretch the
hamstrings.

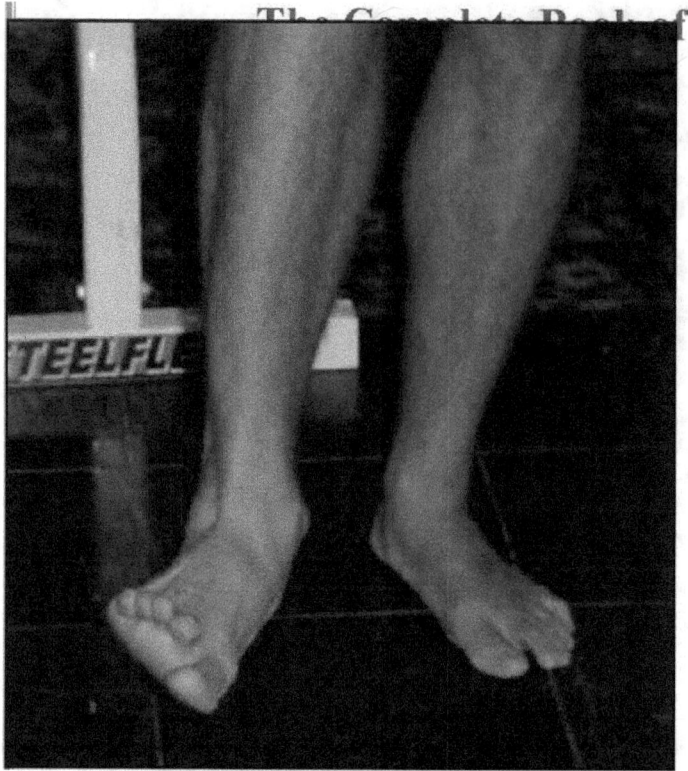

Rotate the ank
them flexible.

Rotate the ankles to keep them flexible.

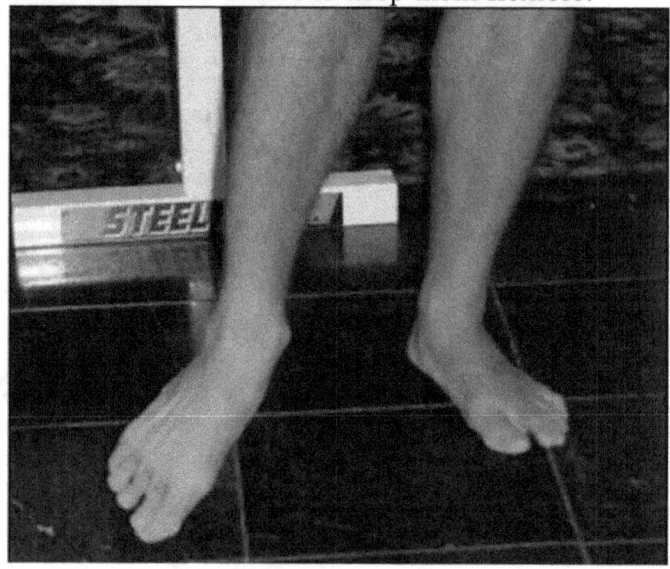

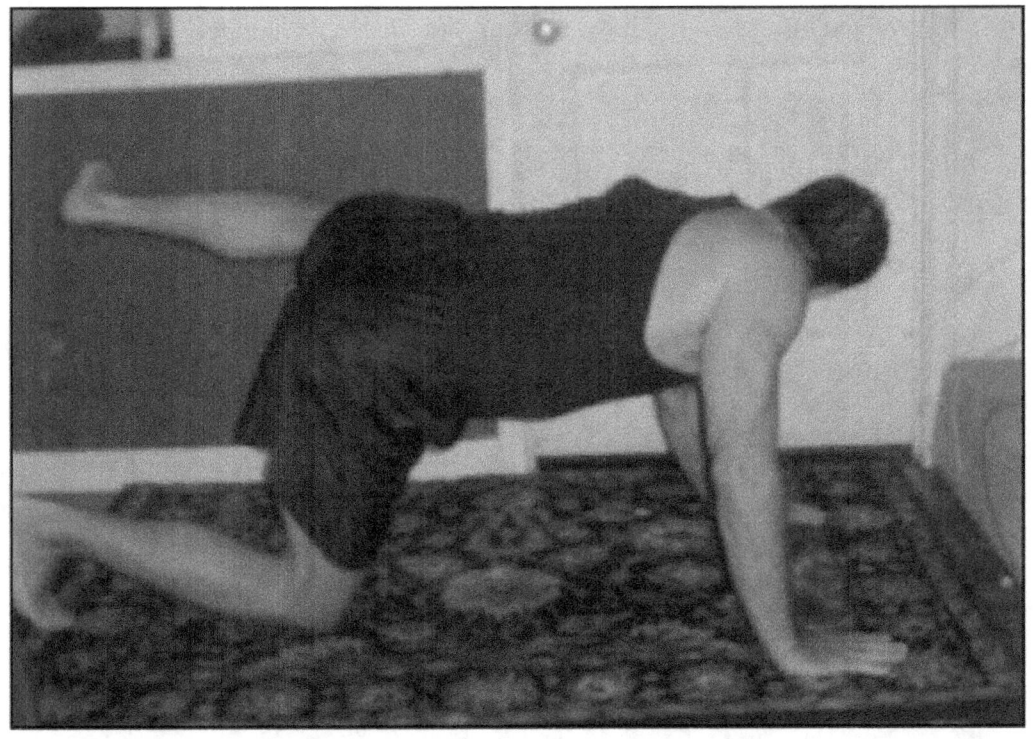

Sit on the hands and knees and then lift the outside leg up.

Sit on the ground and cross the legs, holding onto the knee and gently turning the body.

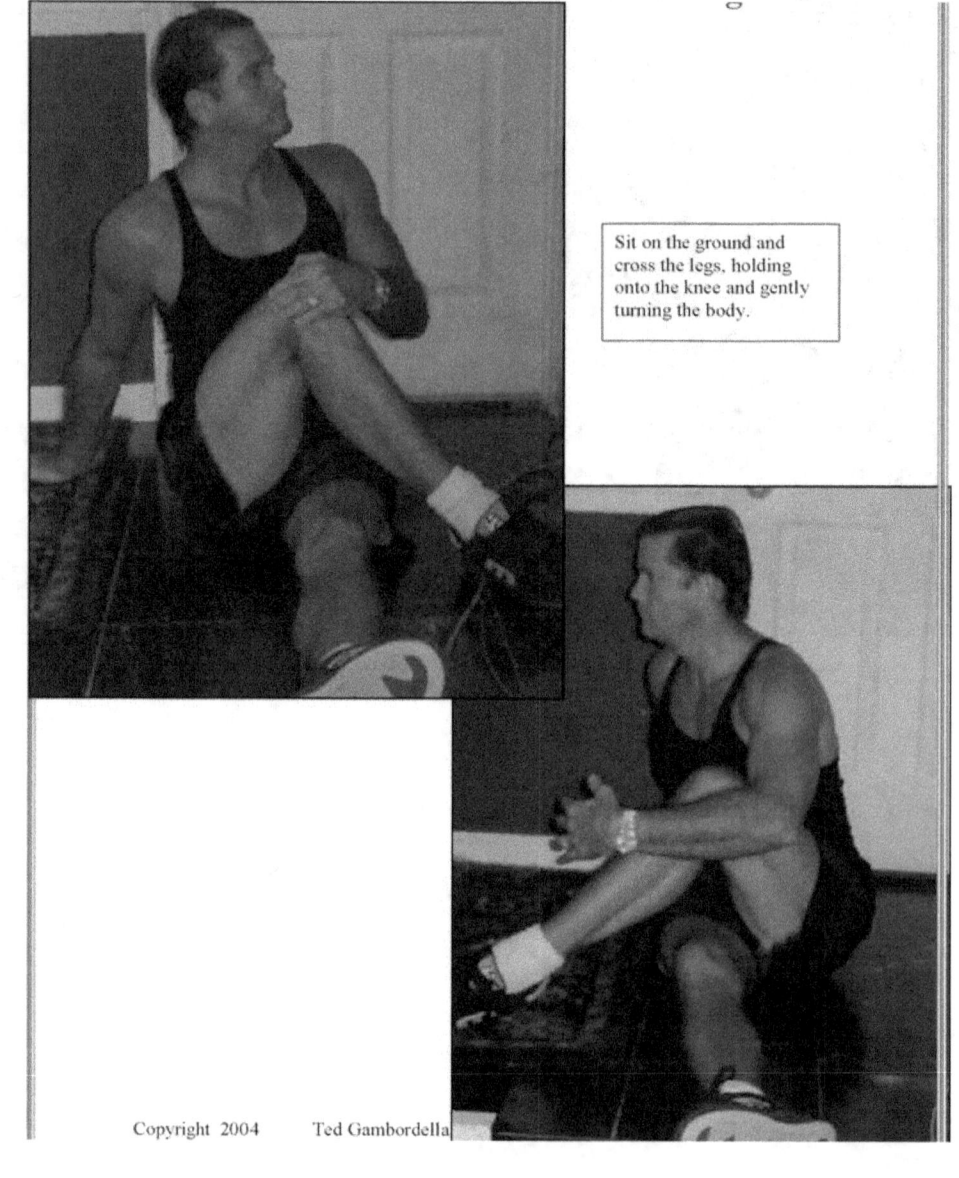

Sit on the ground and cross the legs, holding onto the knee and gently turning the body.

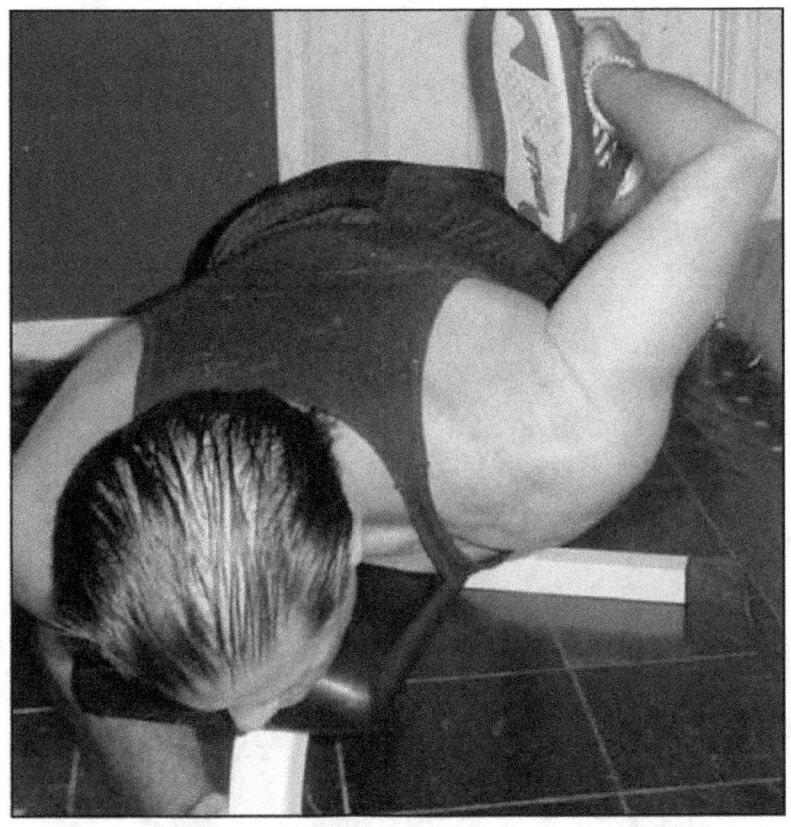

Lie on the bench and reach back and pull the knee to the back.

You can continue this stretch by leaning to the side and pulling on the knee.

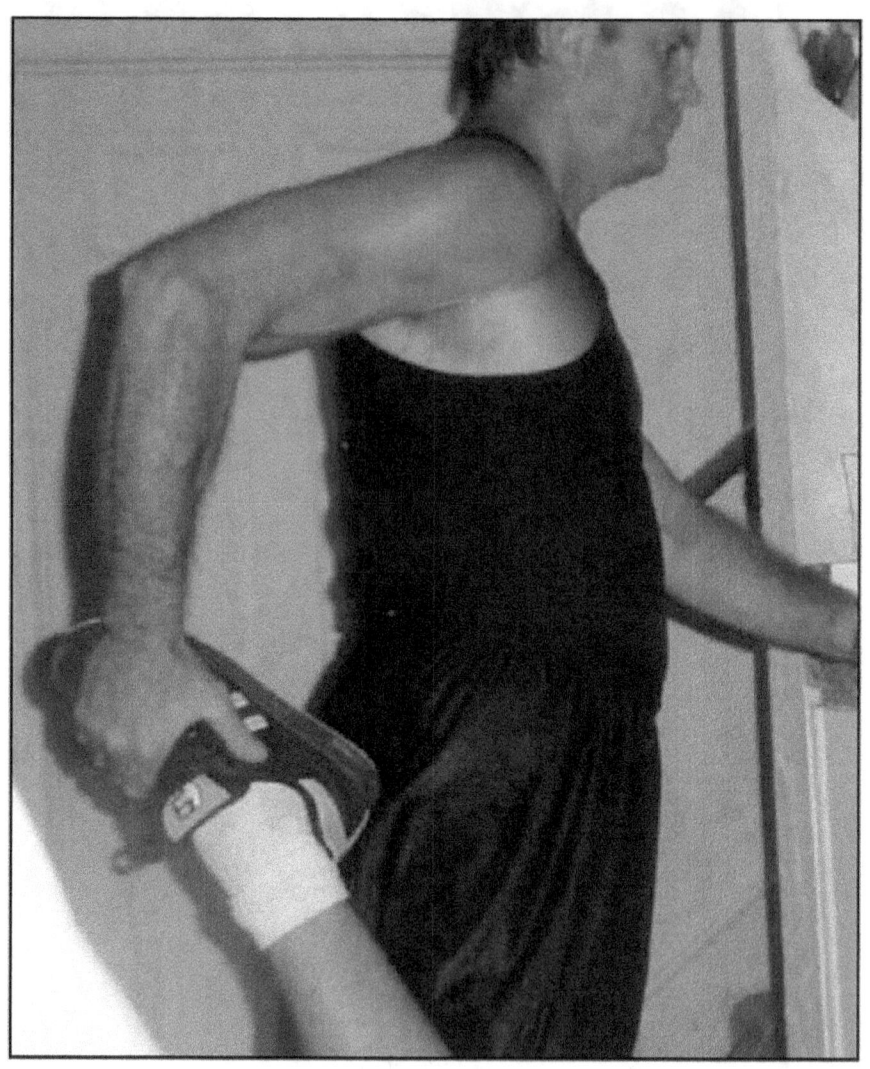

A variation of the hamstring stretch, where you stand and reach back grab the foot and pull it to the buttocks.

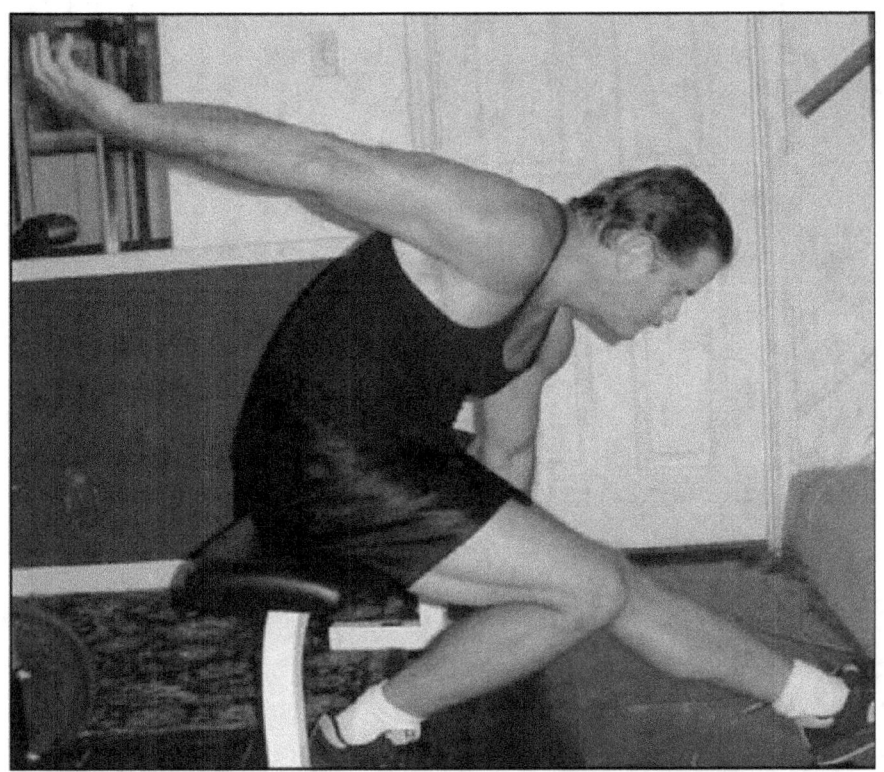

Put one leg straight out while sitting and reach back with the opposite arm. Alternate arms.

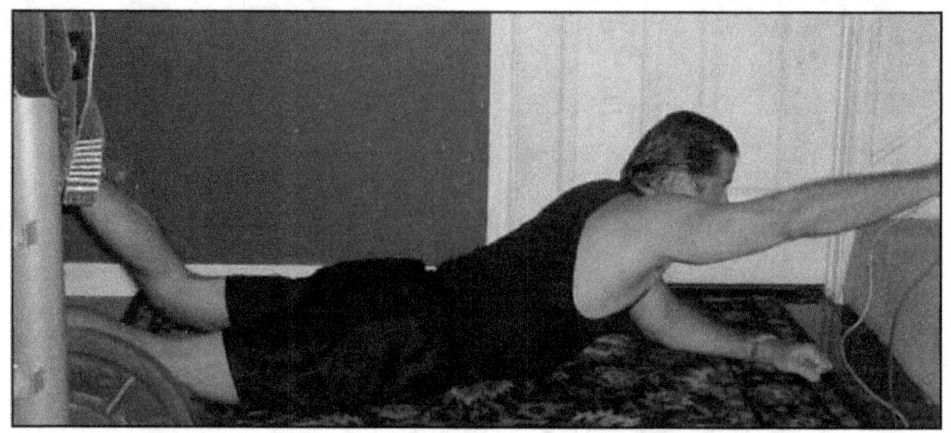

Lie on the stomach and reach one leg back and up and the opposite arm out and stretch.

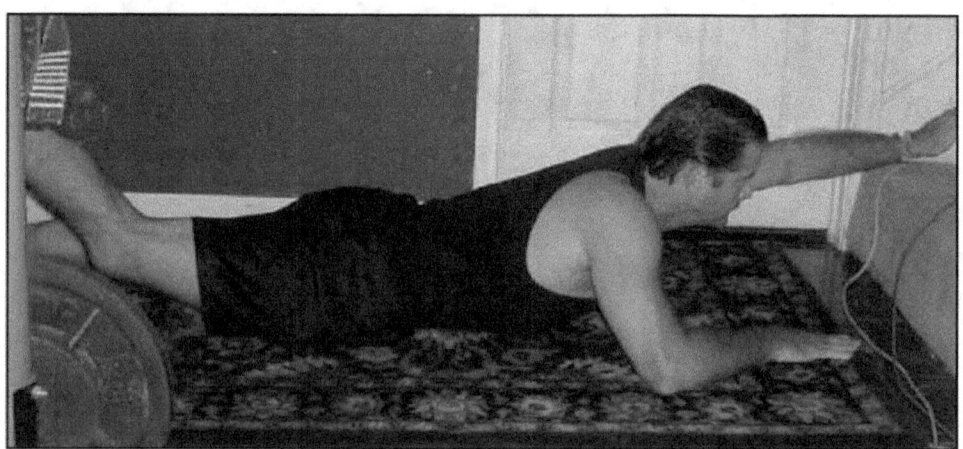

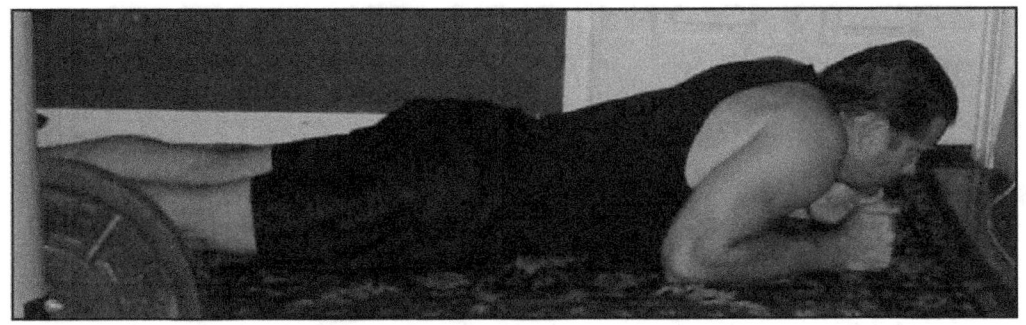

Lie on the elbows and then press the body up to arch the back and stretch it.

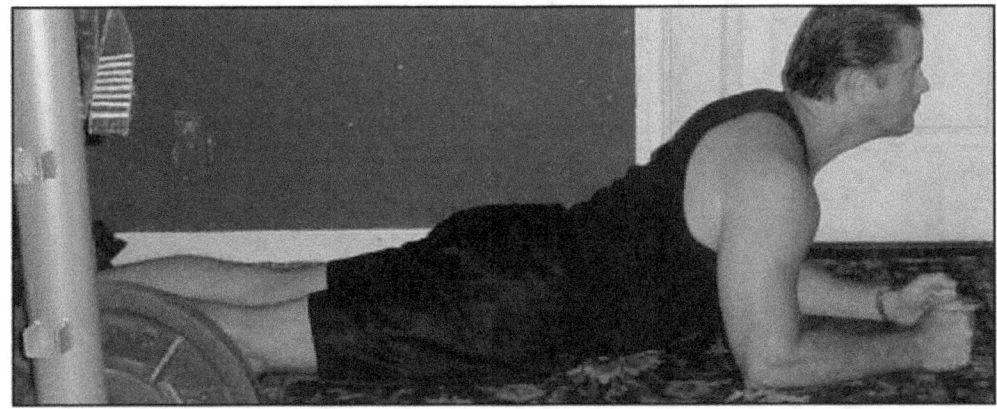

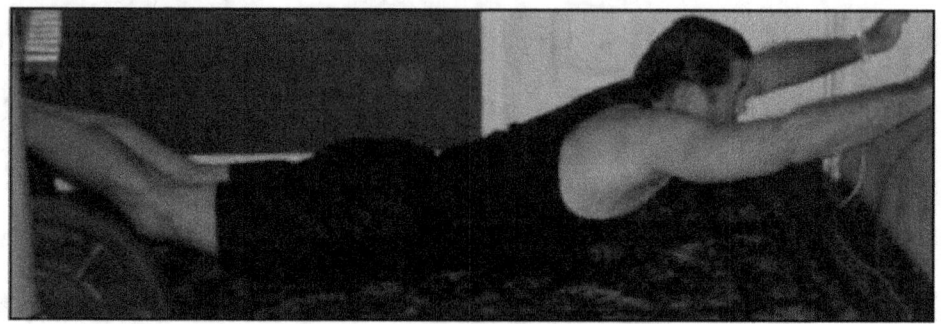

Lie on the stomach and arch the back up, lifting the legs and arms. You can also do it with the arms behind the back.

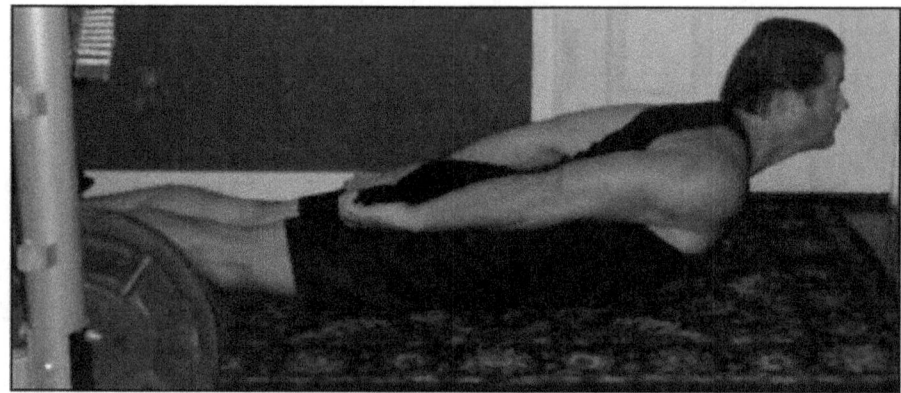

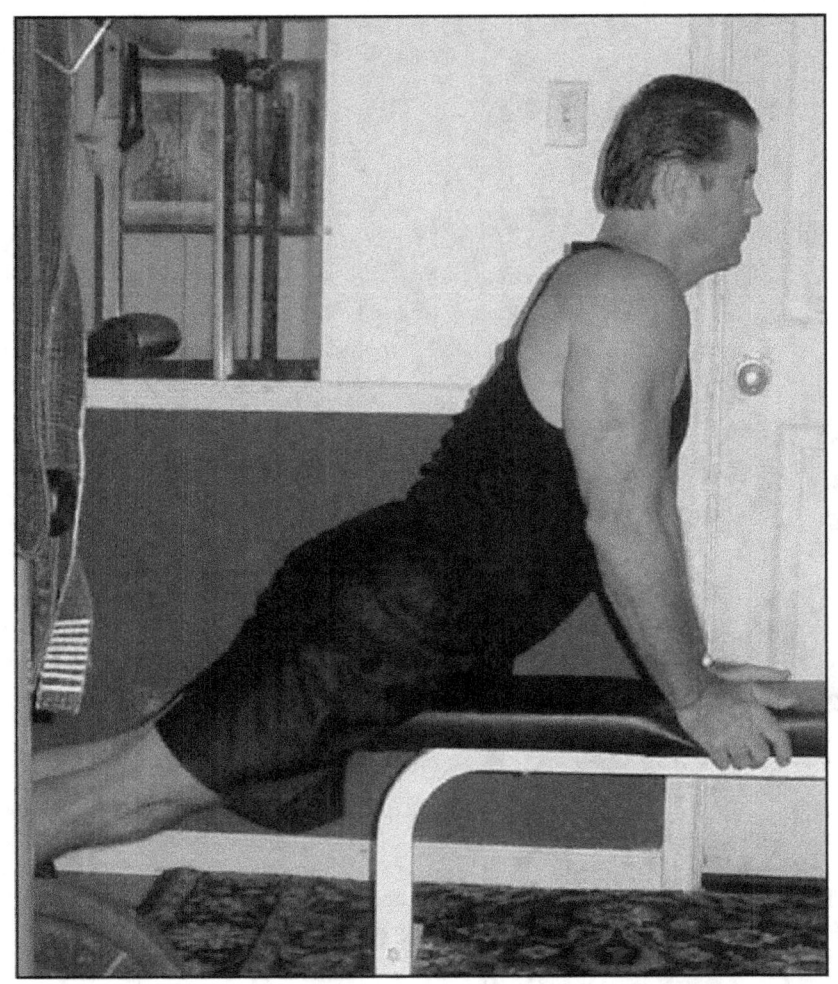

Lean against the bench and place the arms on
it firmly then arch the back up and stretch it.

Lean against the bench
and place the arms on it
firmly then arch the back
up and stretch it.

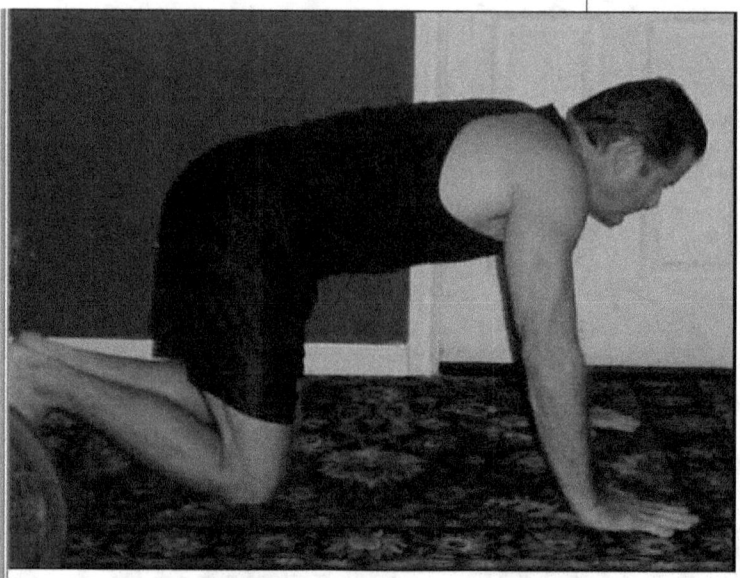

Sit on the hands
and knees and
stretch the back
by arching it up
like a cat
stretching. .

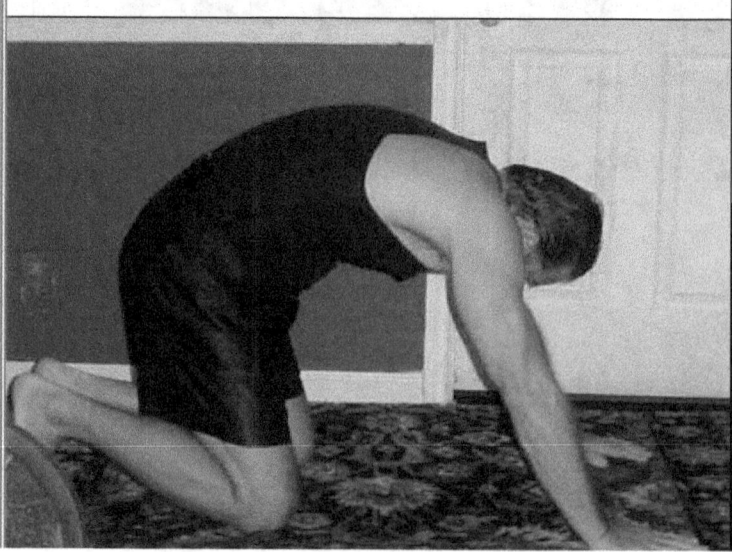

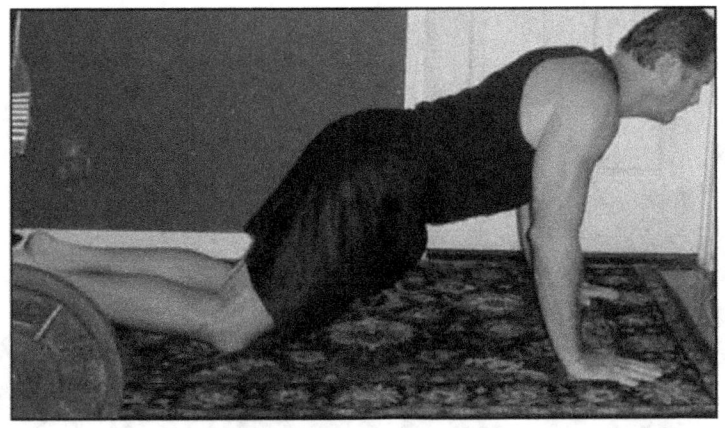

Sit on the hands and knees and then lean forward gently to stretch the back.

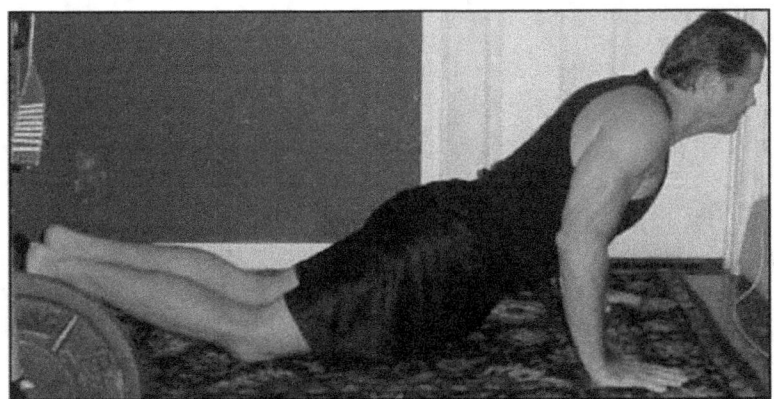

Sit on the hands and knees and put one arm out and the opposite leg back.

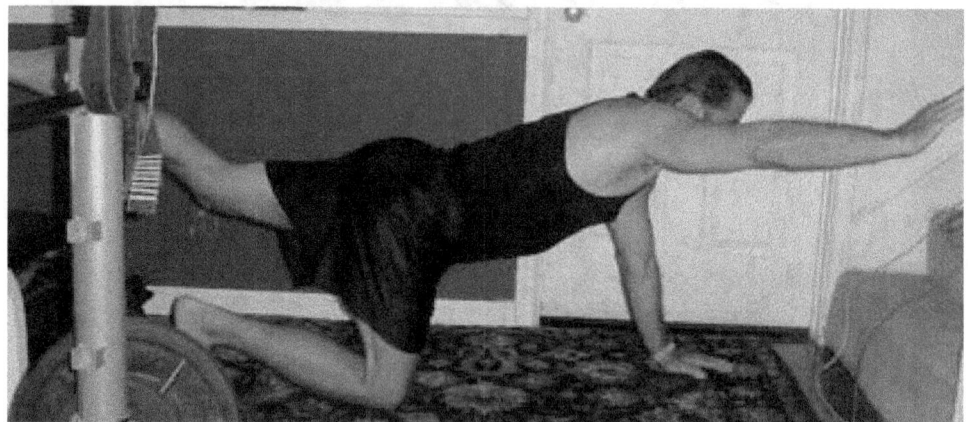

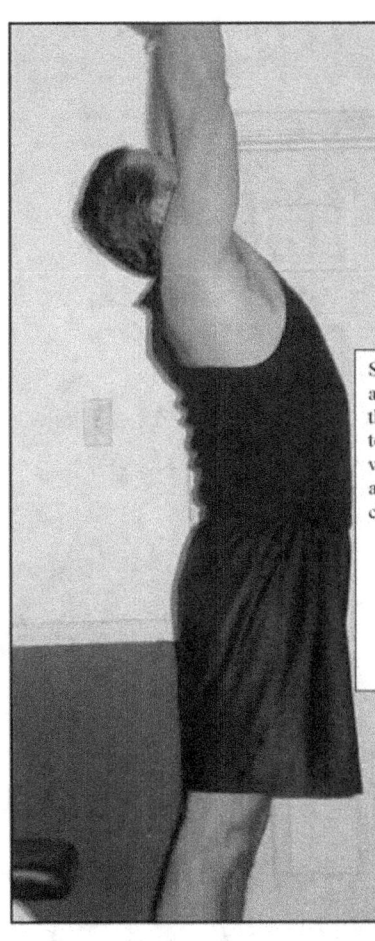

Stand very tall
and reach up,
then stretch up
to the toes
while reaching
as high as you
can.

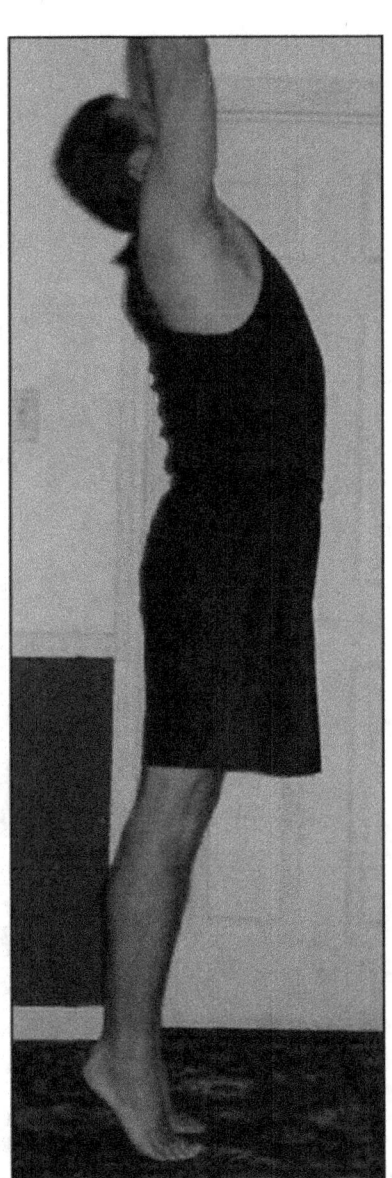

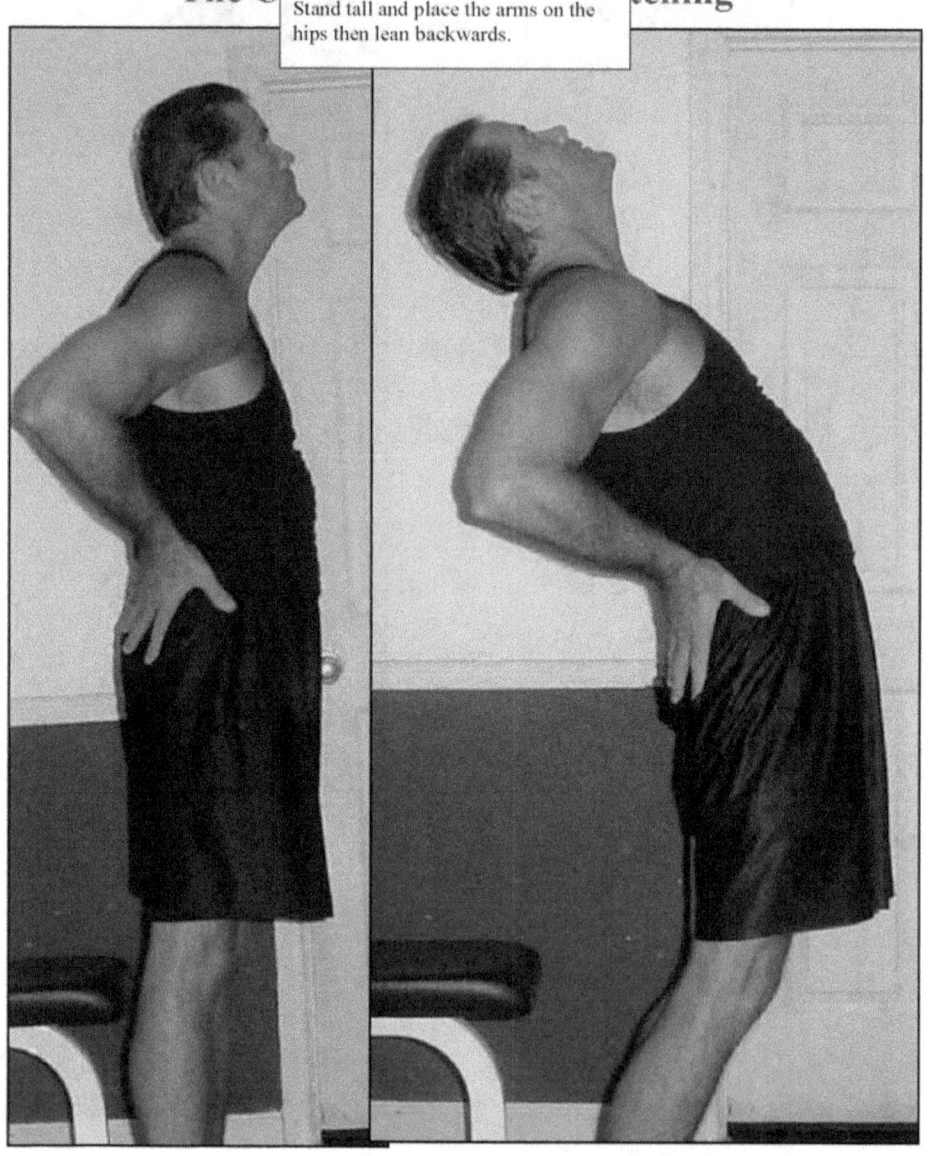

Stand tall and place the arms on the hips then lean backwards.

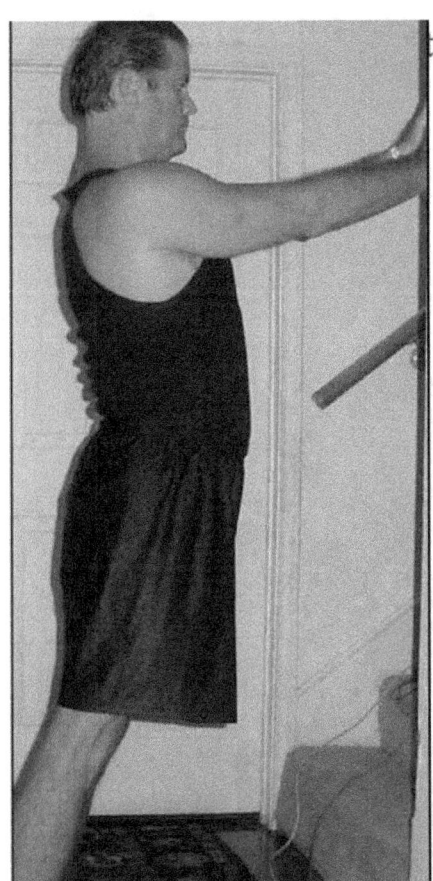

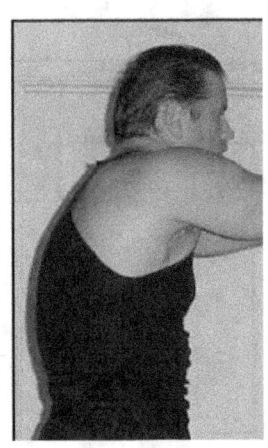

Stand straight and lean agai
the wall, then arch the back
away from the wall.

Stand straight and lean against
the wall, then arch the back
away from the wall.

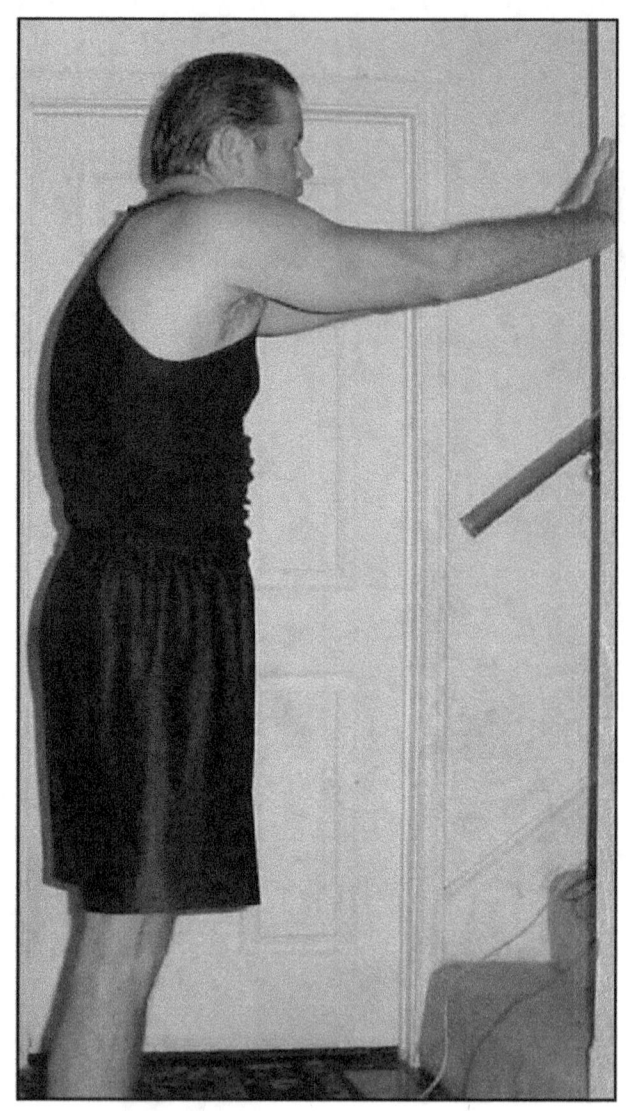

Lean over against the bench and twist the body to the right and left.

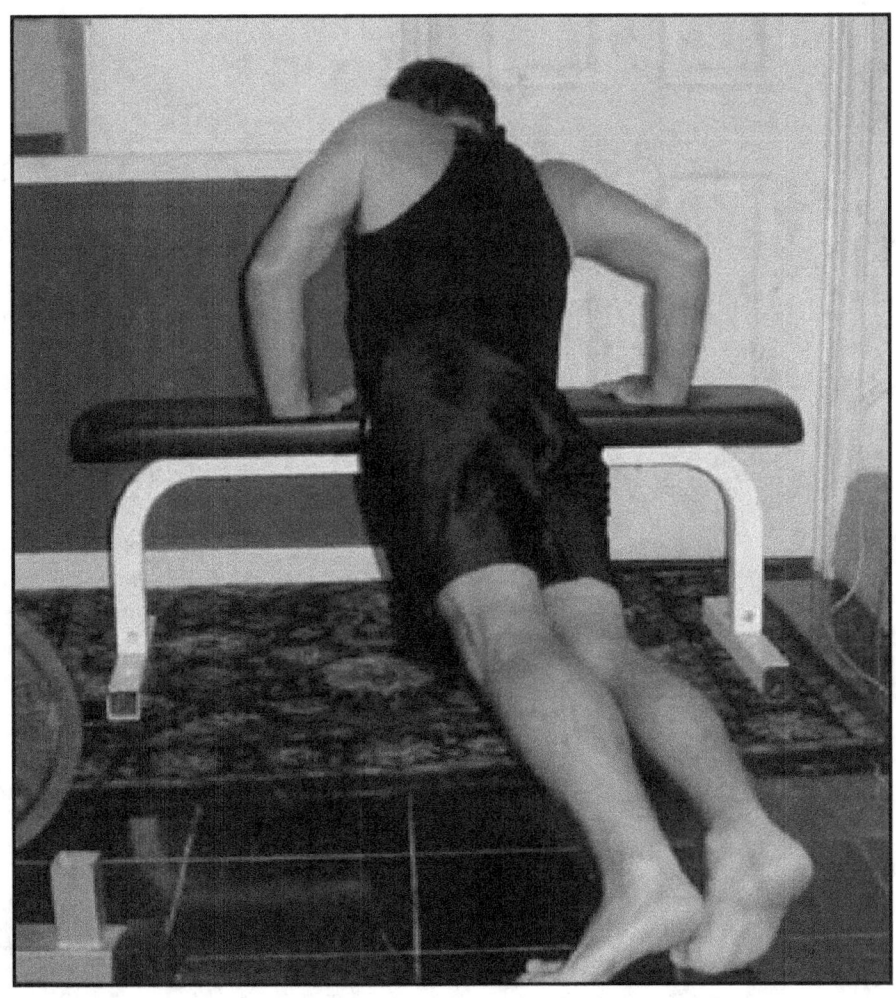

Reach down and let the body relax to touch the toes.

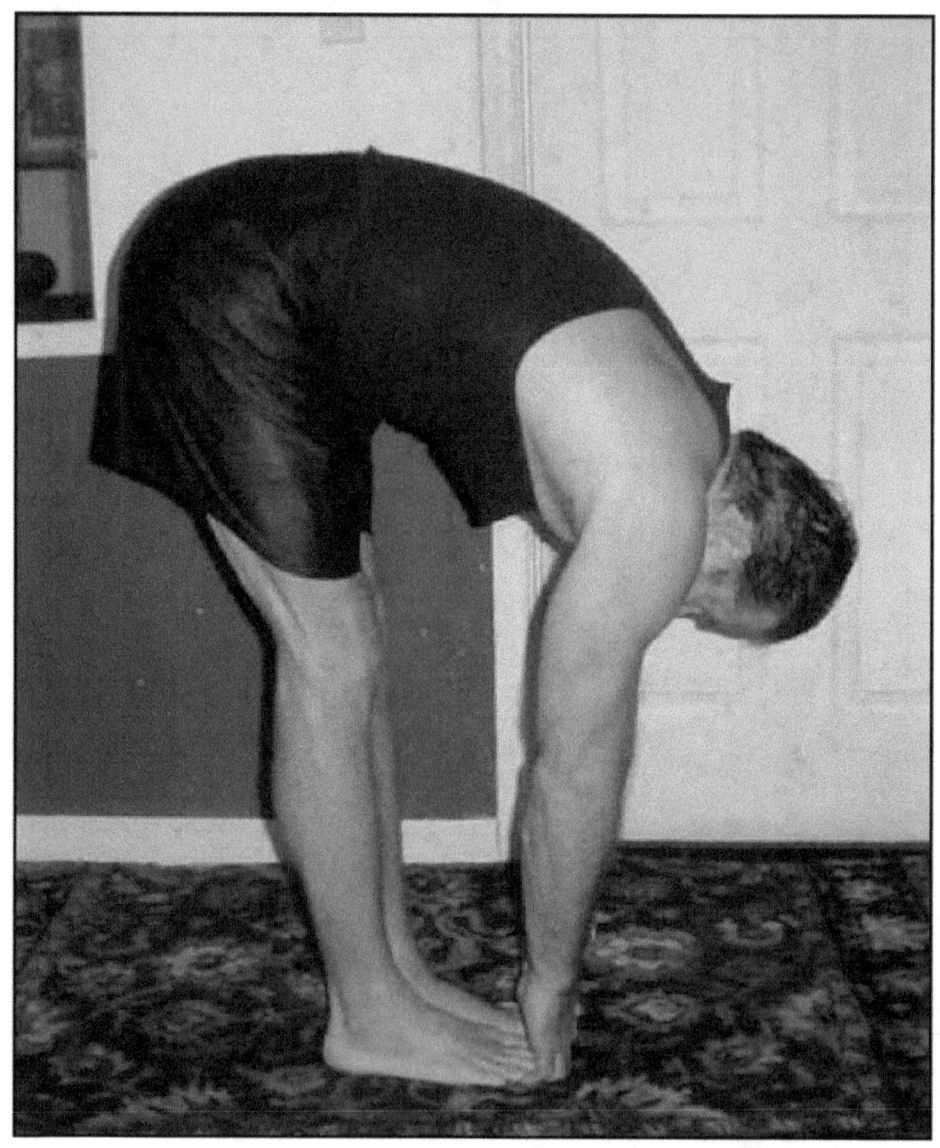

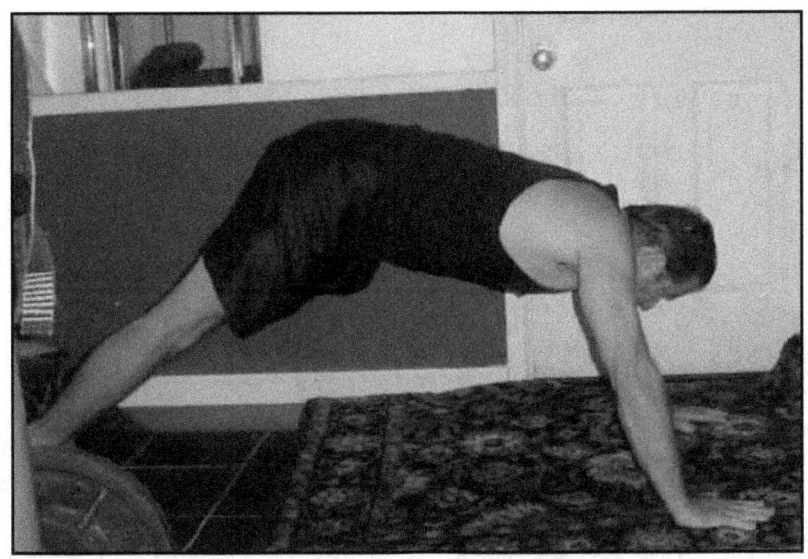

Start by arching the back high from the hand and toes, then drop down to relax.

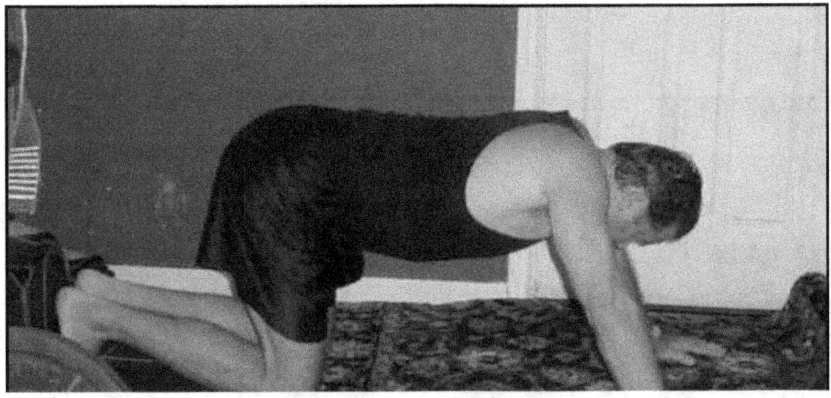

Start by arching the back high from the hand and toes, then drop down to relax.

Arch the body up and then drop it down supported by the hands and toes.

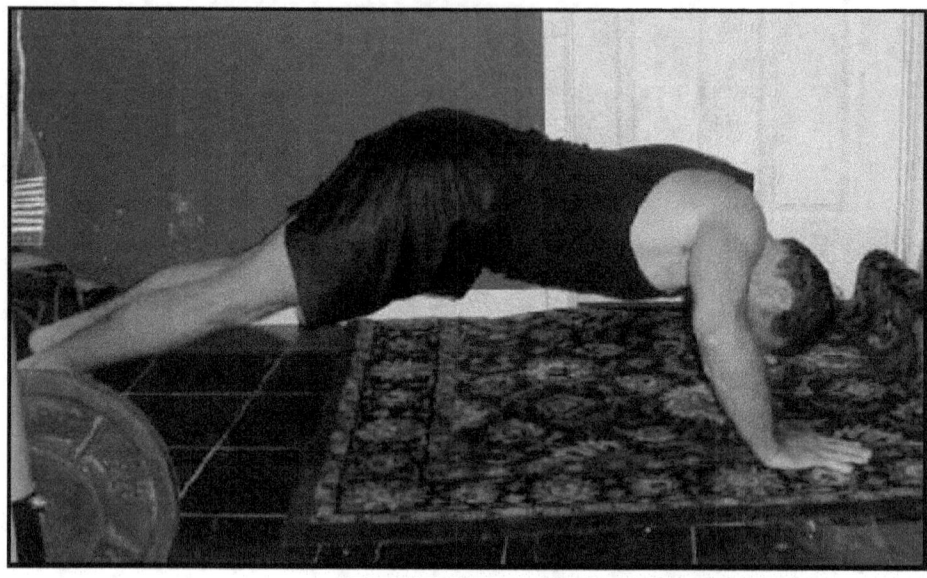

Arch the body up and then drop it down
supported by the hands and toes.

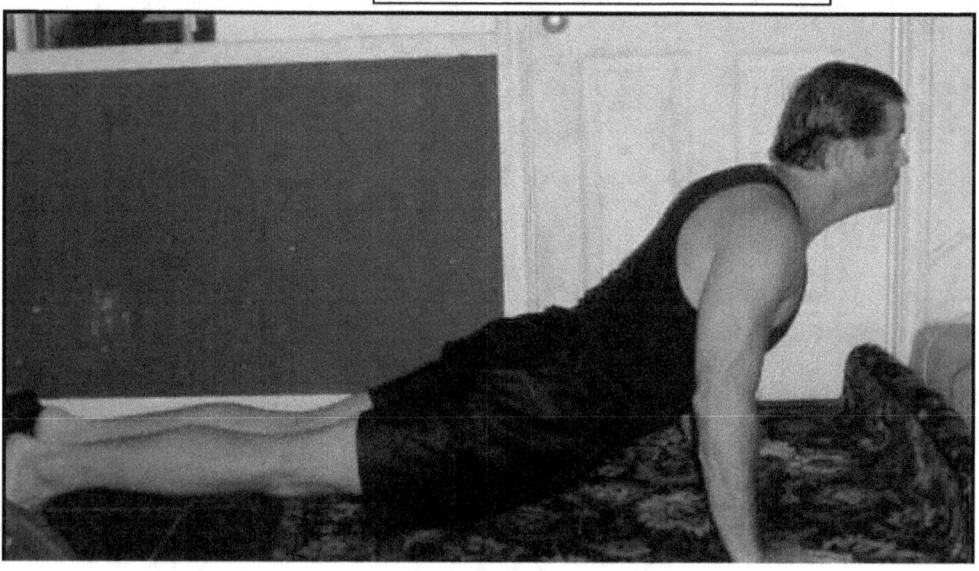

The basic body twist is done by placing the hands on the hips and gently twisting from side to side.

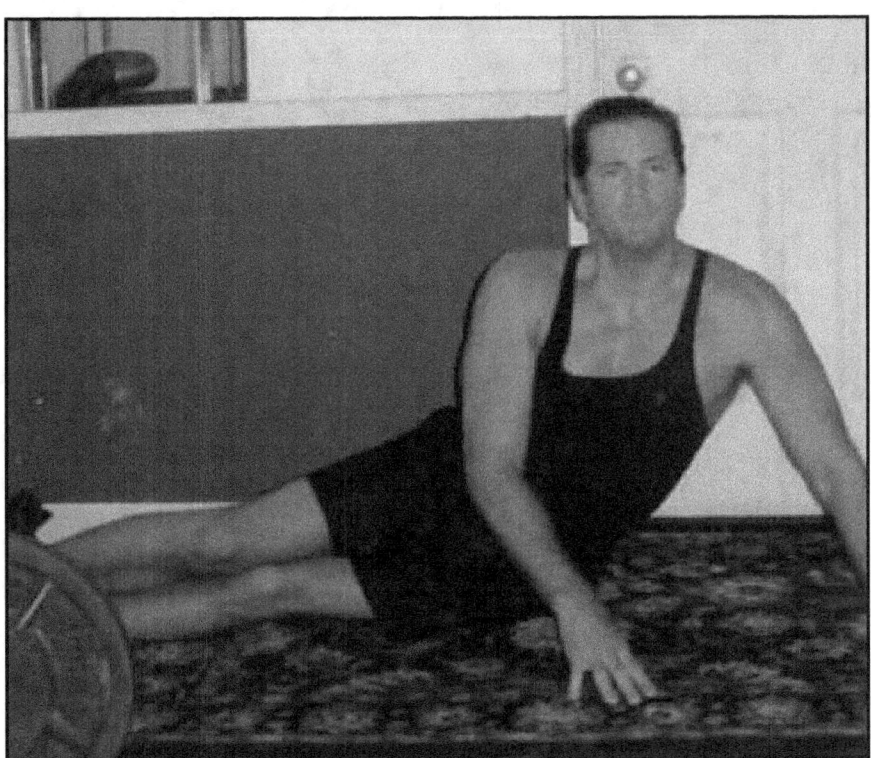

Lie on the floor on your side and then supported by your hands arch the body up to the side.

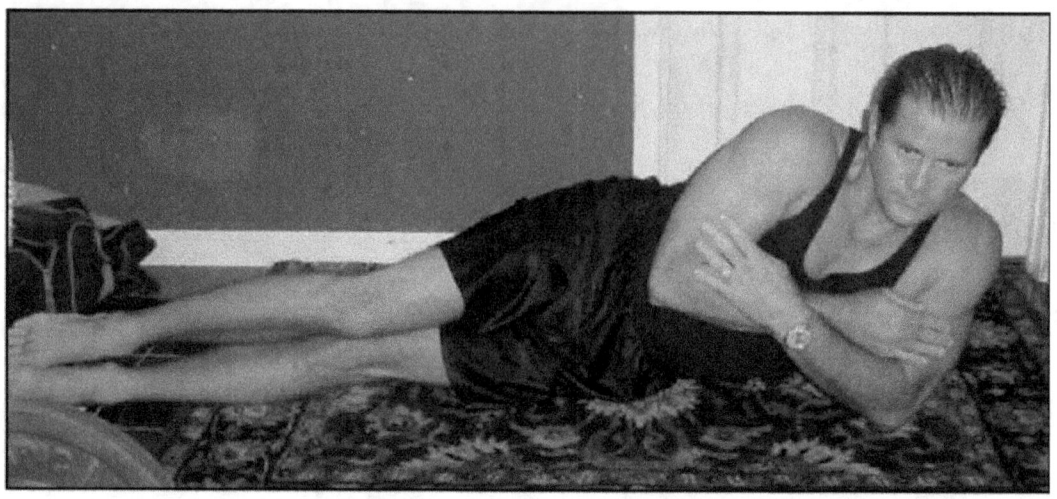

You can also arch the body up to the side with using only the side muscles by crossing the arms.

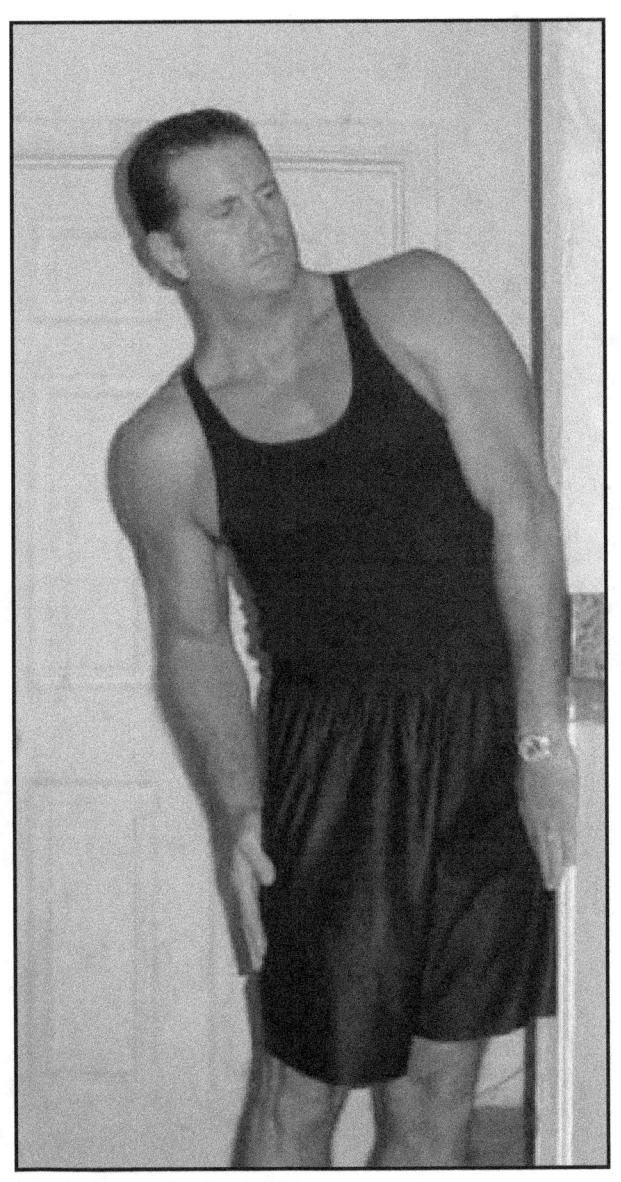

Lean against the wall and arch the body to the side, while keeping the hand on the wall.

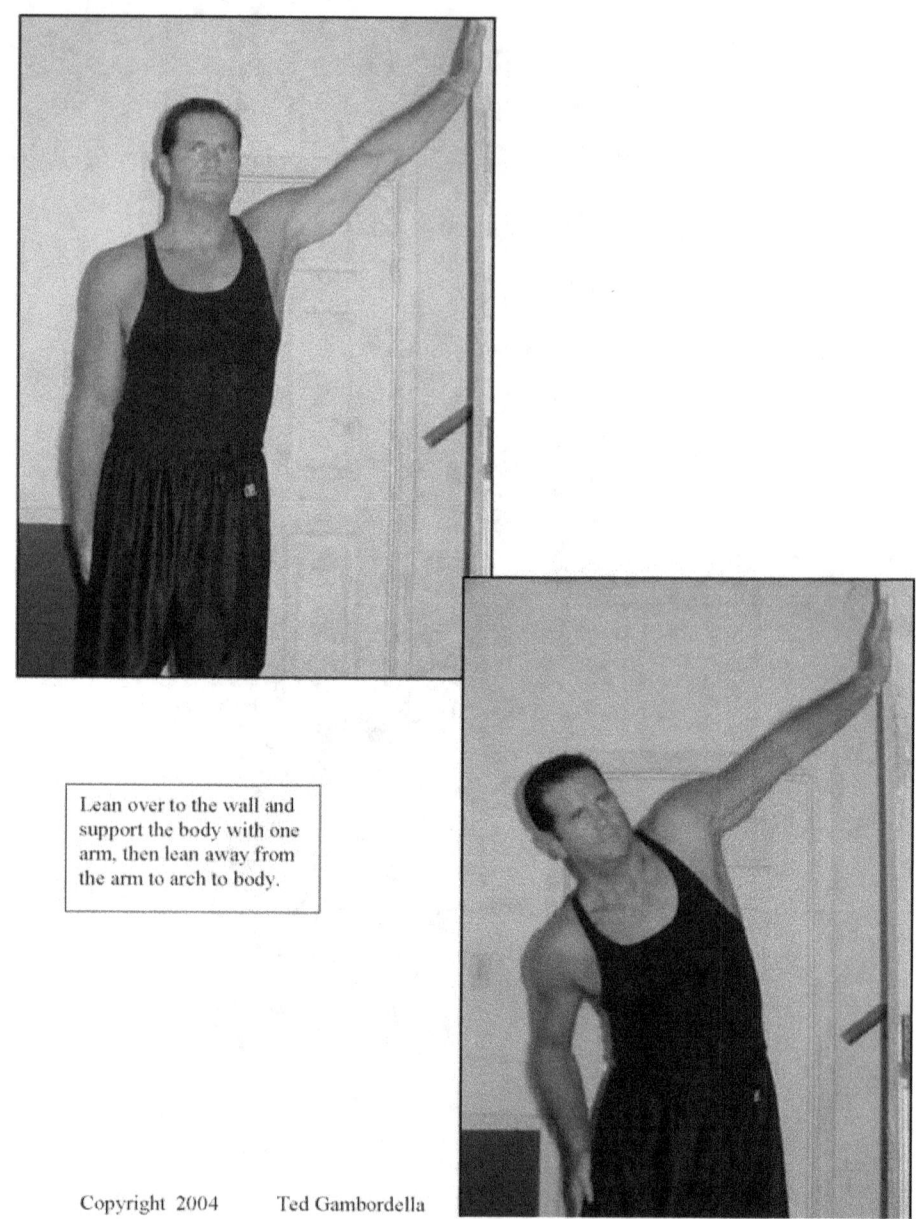

Lean over to the wall and support the body with one arm, then lean away from the arm to arch to body.

Lean over to the wall and support the body with one arm, then lean away from the arm to arch to body.

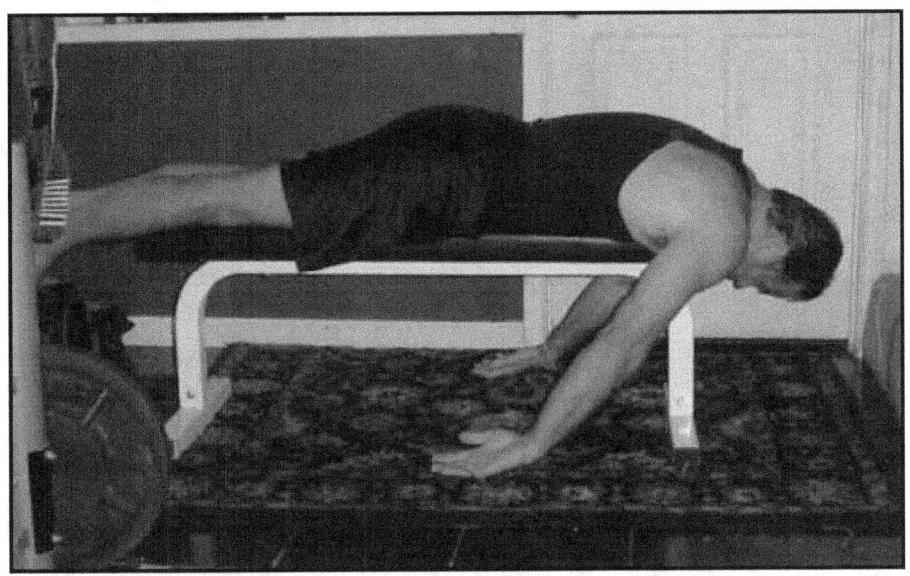

Lie flat on the bench with
the head over the edge and
relax, then slowly reach
up and back with one arm.

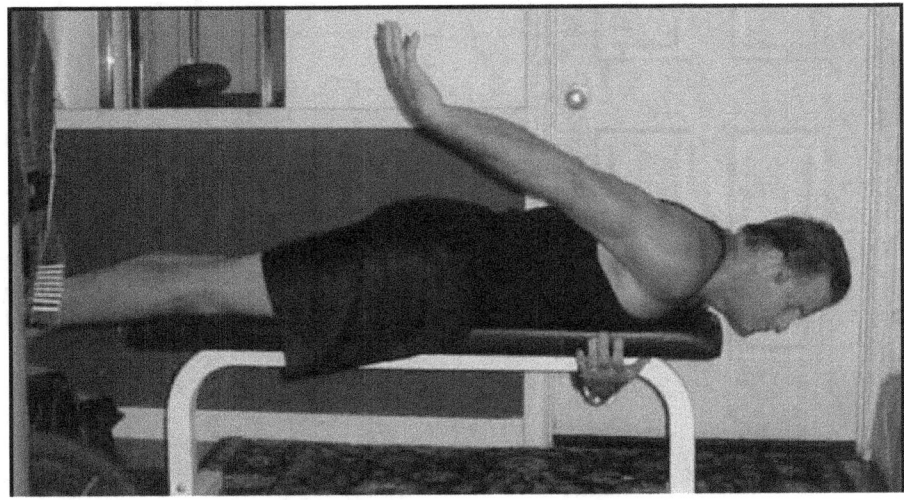

Lie flat on the bench with the head over the edge and relax, then slowly reach up and back with one arm.

Neck Stretches

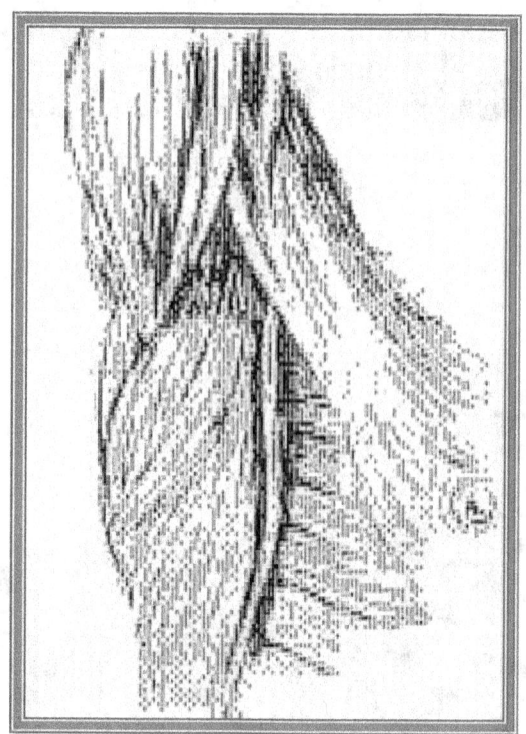

Do all stretches 6 to 8 times. Relax and breath easy, do not bounce or force the stretch..

Place the fist against the neck and gently press it to the right and then to the left.

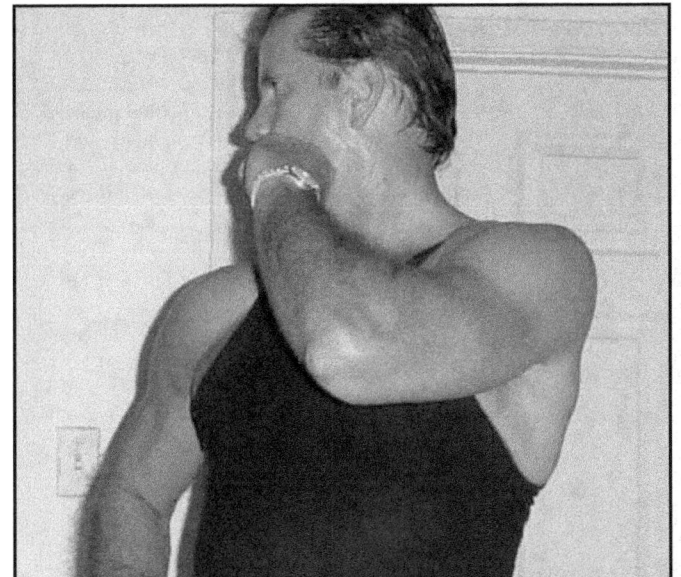

Place the fist against the neck and gently press it to the right and then to the left.

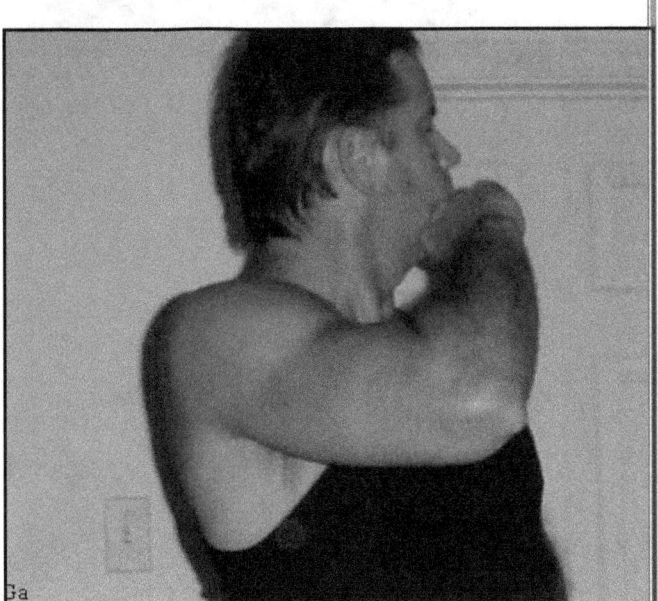

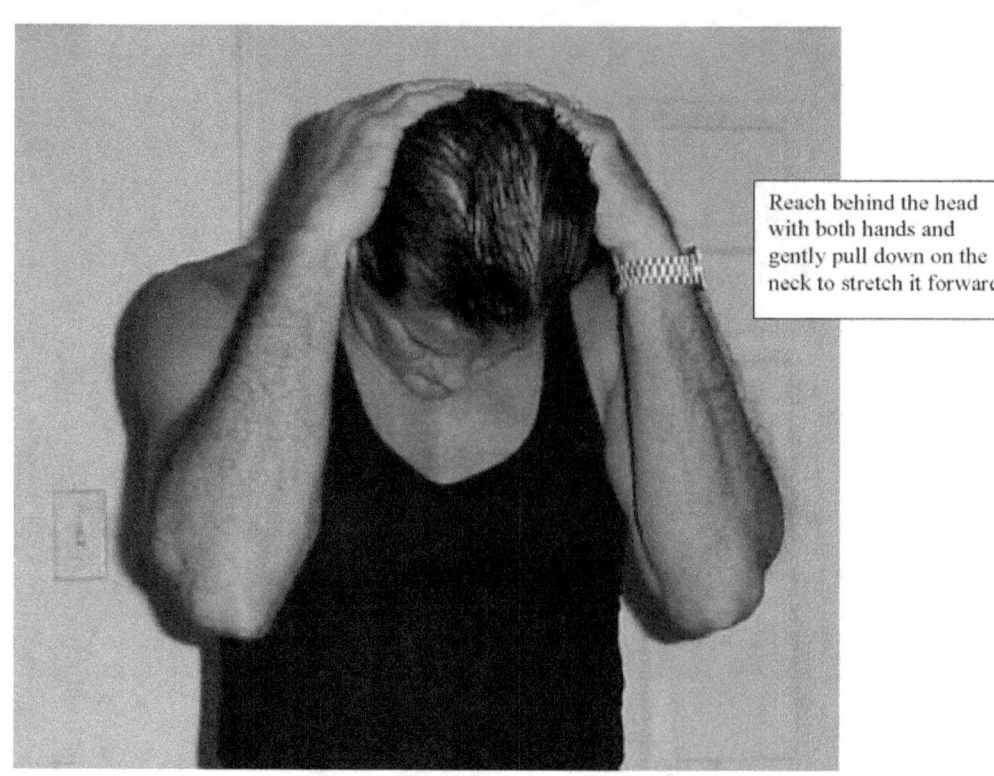

Reach behind the head with both hands and gently pull down on the neck to stretch it forward.

Neck circles. Hold the arms on the hips and gently rotate the neck in circles, first clockwise then counter clockwise

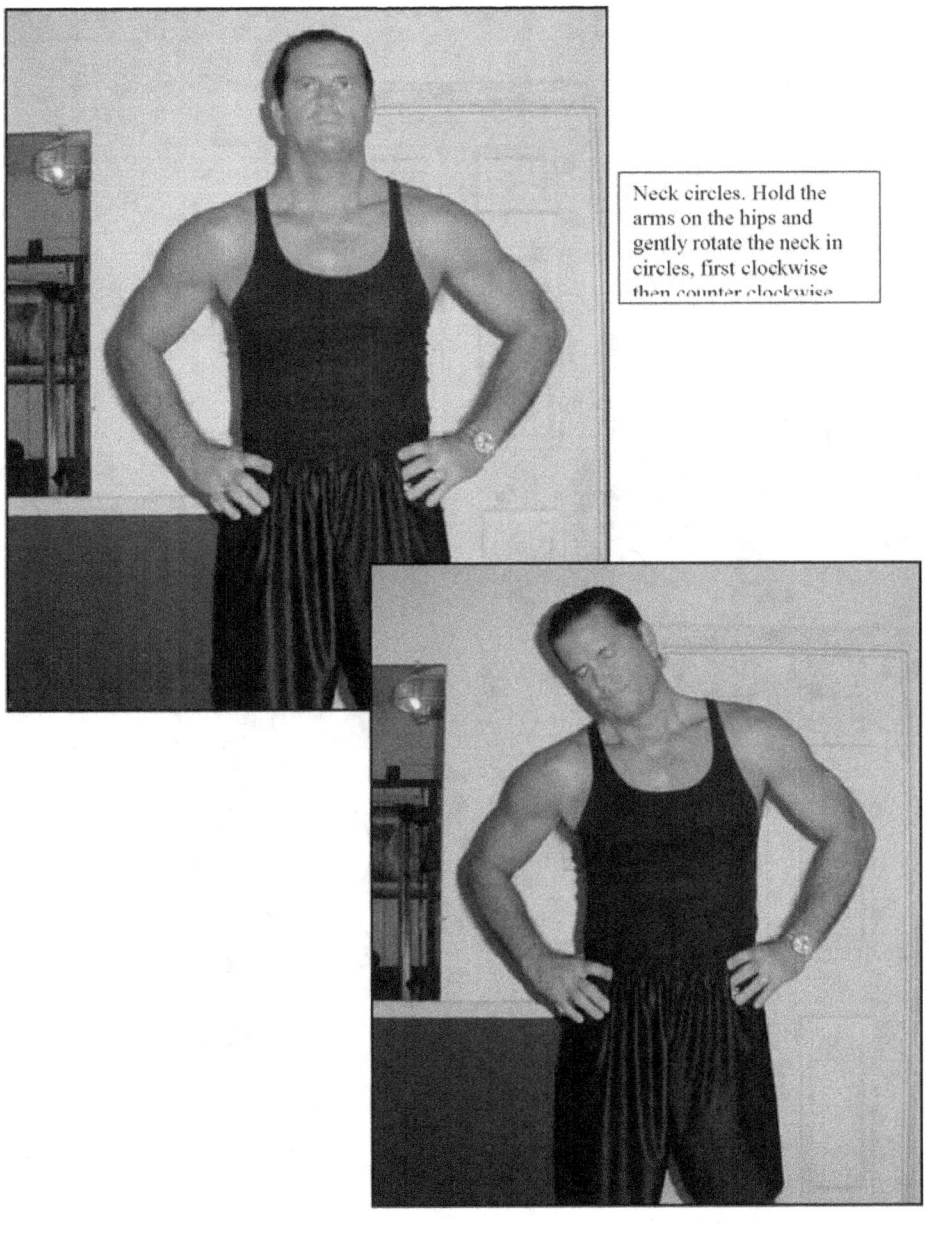

Neck circles. Hold the arms on the hips and gently rotate the neck in circles, first clockwise then counter clockwise

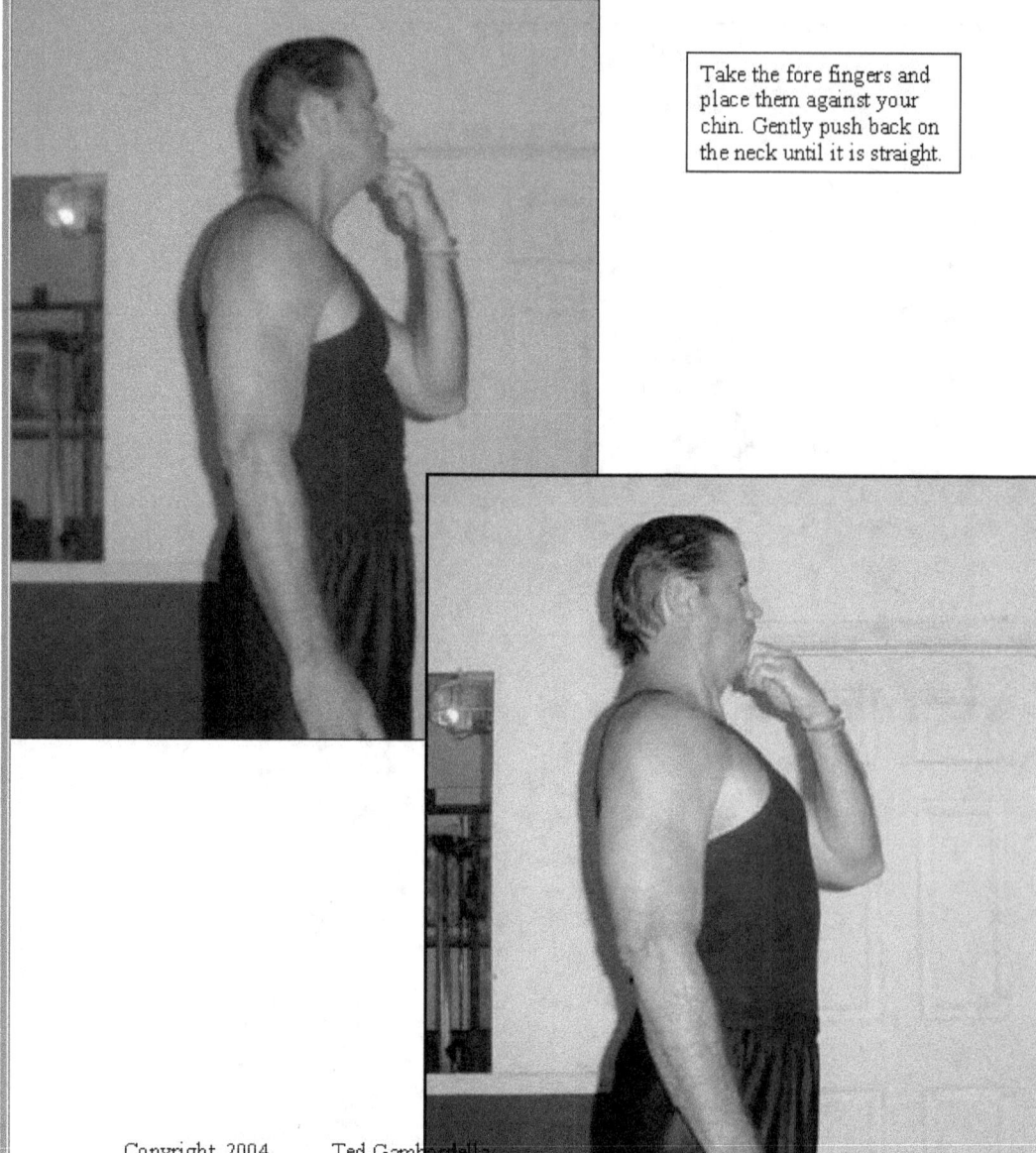

Take the fore fingers and place them against your chin. Gently push back on the neck until it is straight.

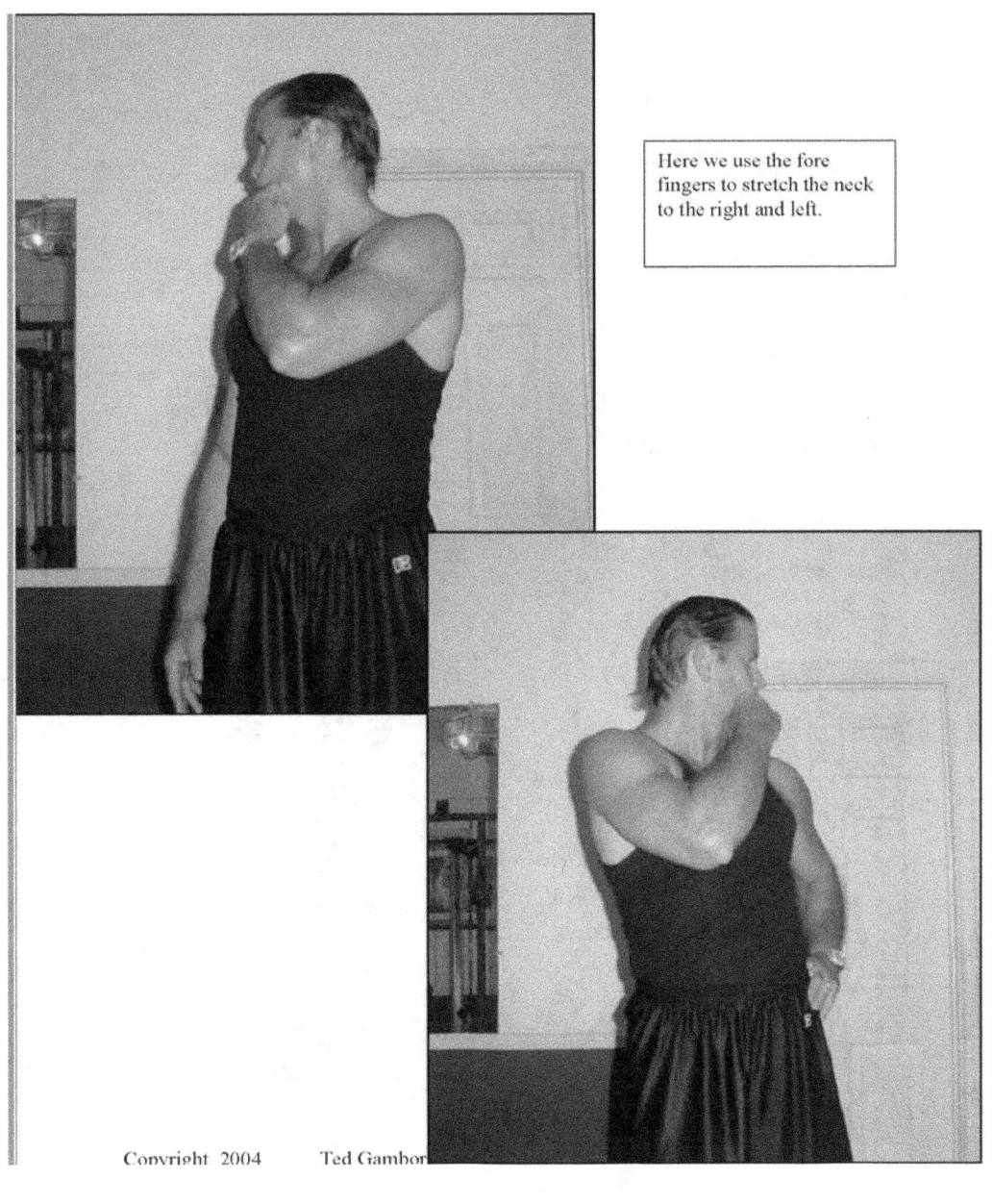

Here we use the fore
fingers to stretch the neck
to the right and left.

Cross both hands behind the neck and gently pull down on the neck to

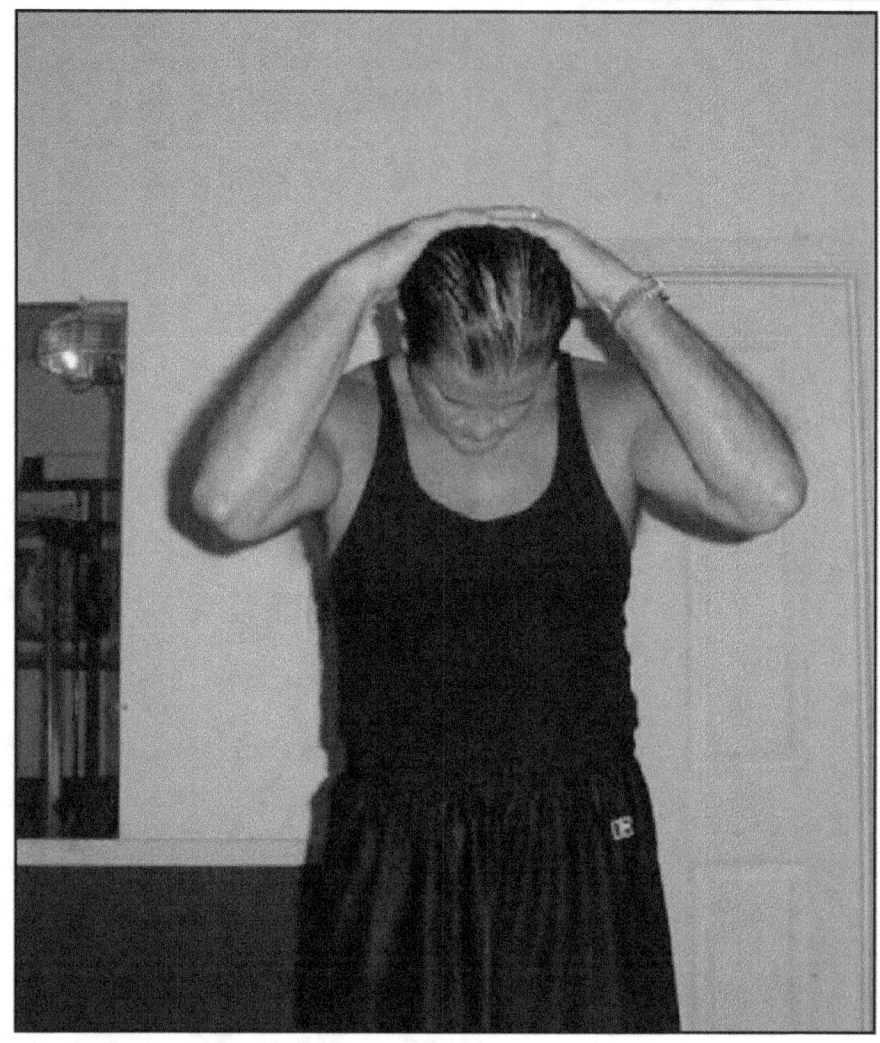

Here we stretch the neck backwards by placing both of our hands under the jaw.

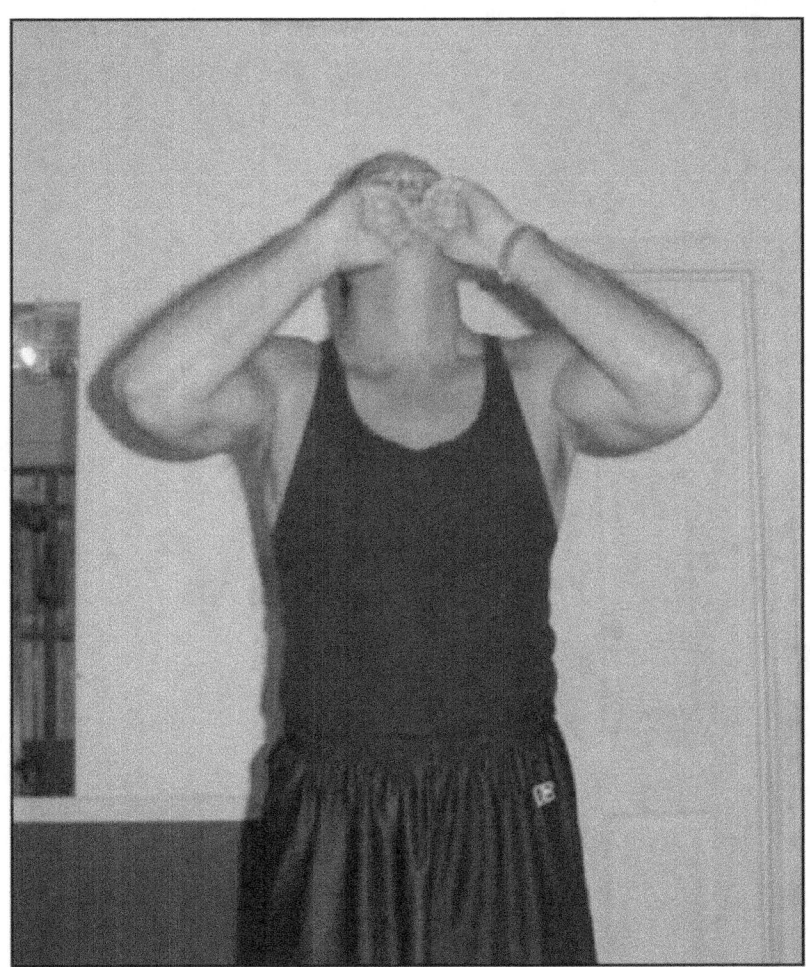

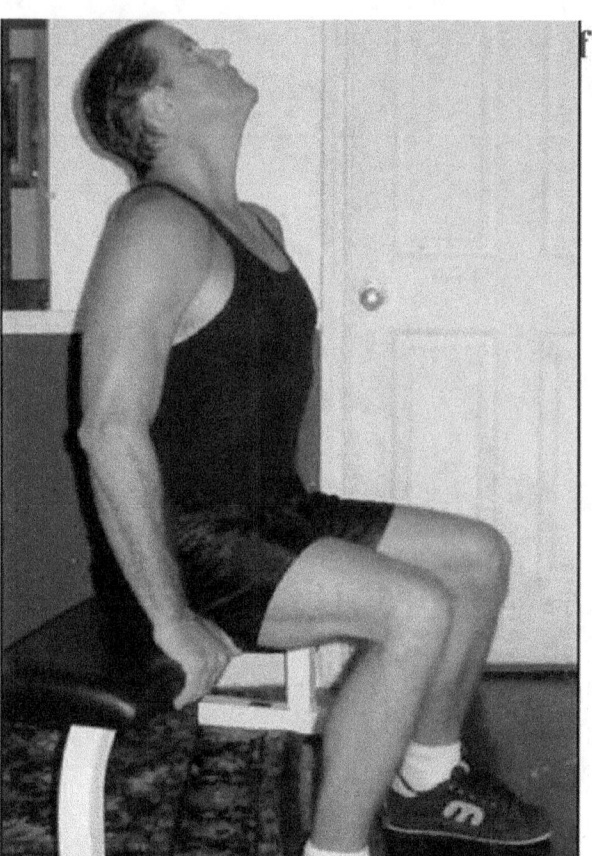

Sit on a bench or a chair and keeping the back straight pull the head and neck back as far a possible.

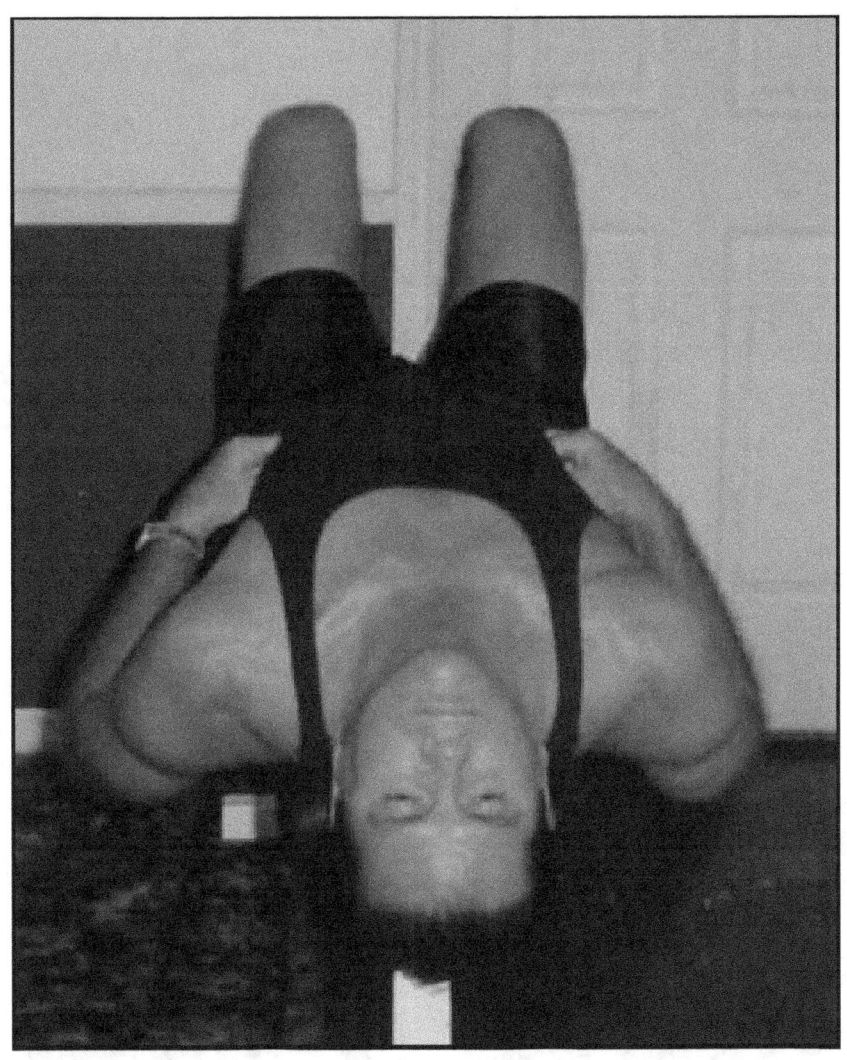

Let your body hand over the edge of the bench and then relax the neck by letting it stretch.

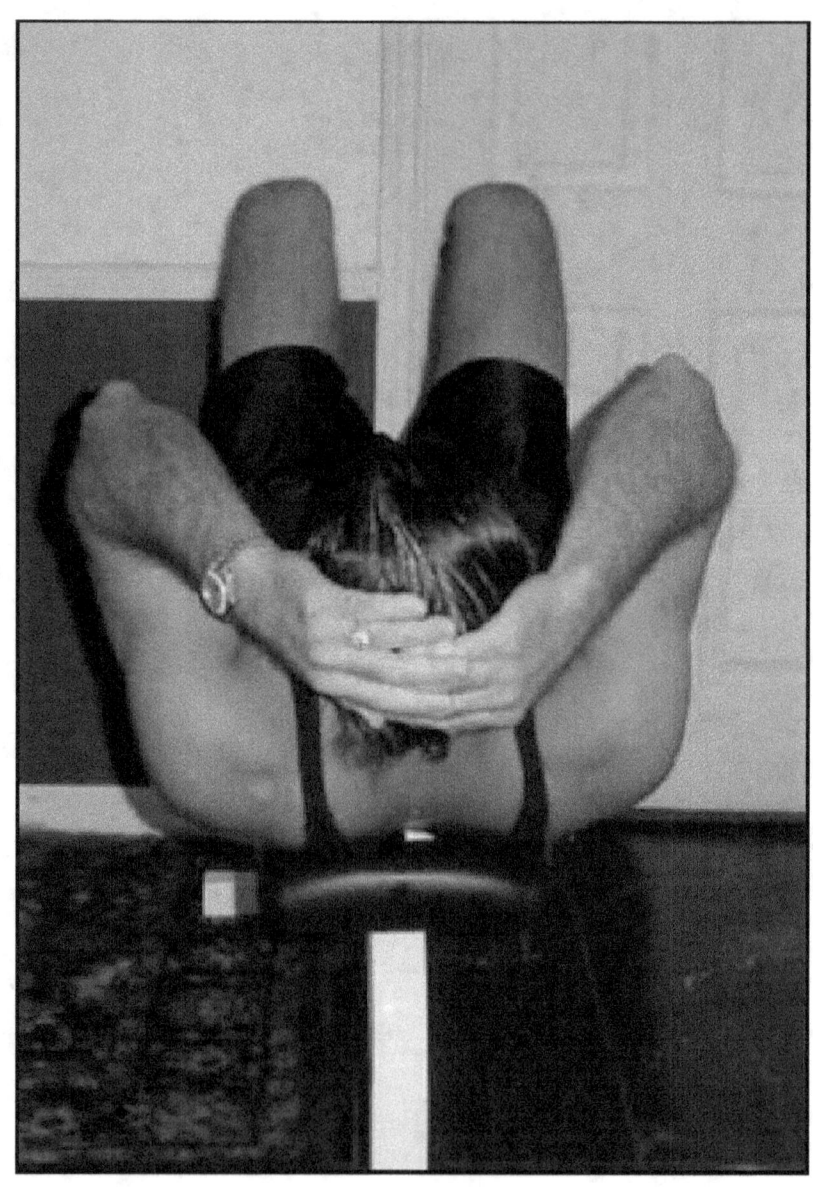

After the neck has relaxed, reach down and pull gently up on the neck.
Here we practice good posture by sitting hunched over and then pulling the body
back and keeping the neck in a straight line.

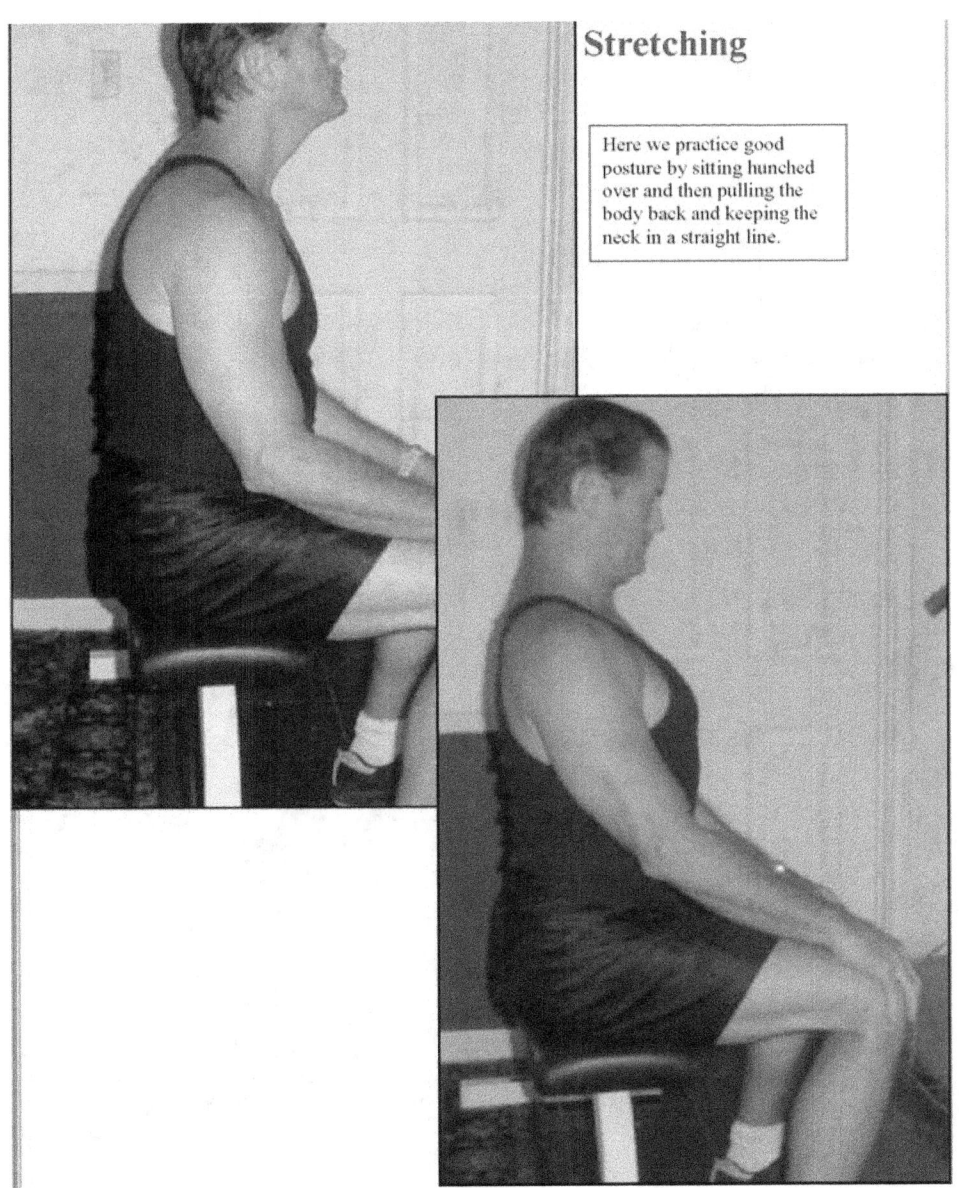

Stretching

Here we practice good posture by sitting hunched over and then pulling the body back and keeping the neck in a straight line.

Place the arms on the back of the neck and flex them to stretch the chest and shoulders.

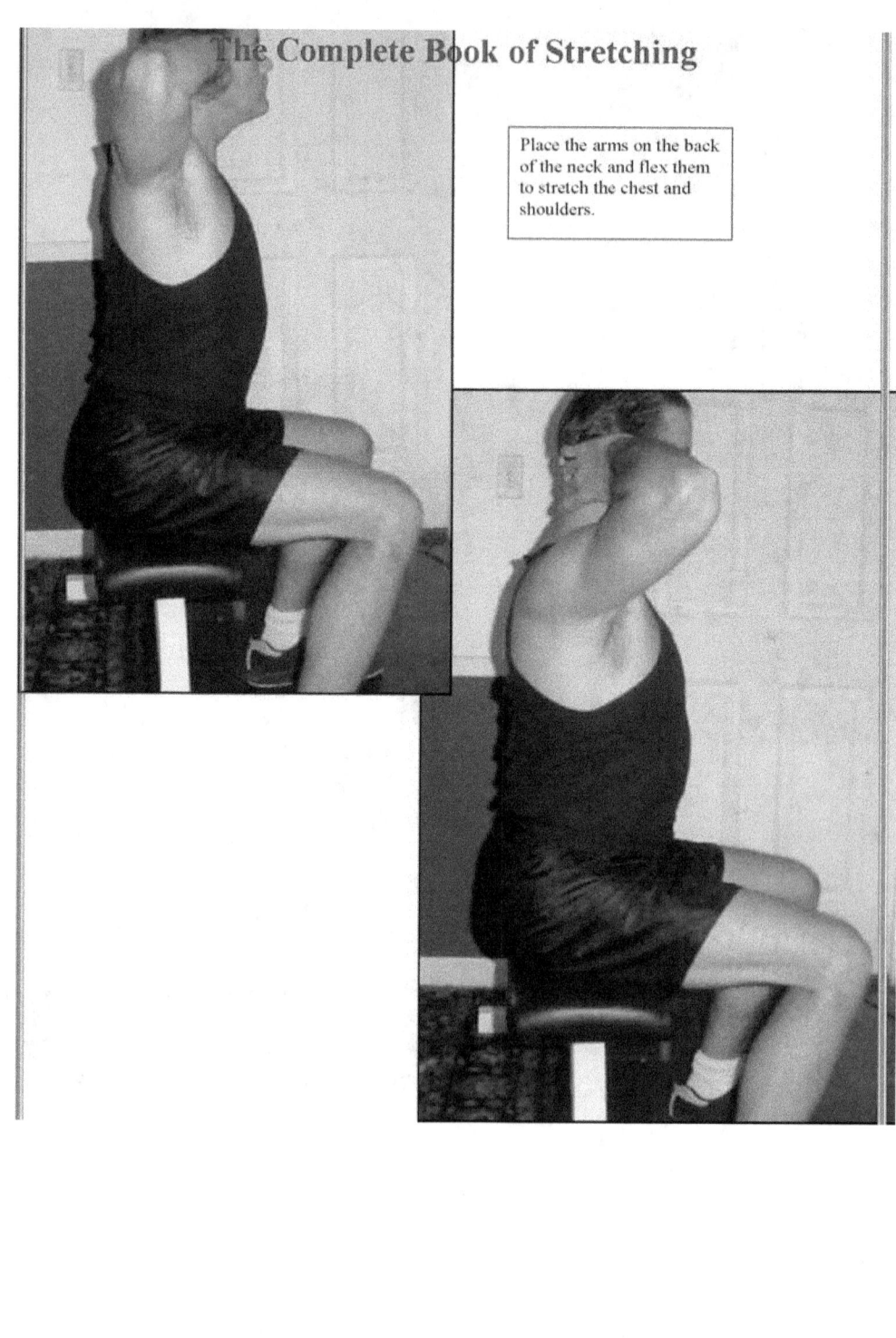

Place the arms on the back of the neck and flex them to stretch the chest and shoulders.

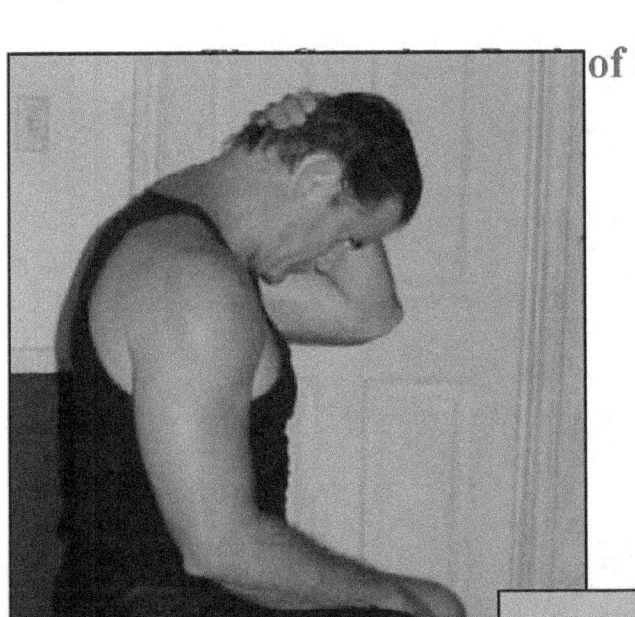

Reach up and grab the back of your neck and pull the head down and then gently resist as you pull the head backwards. .

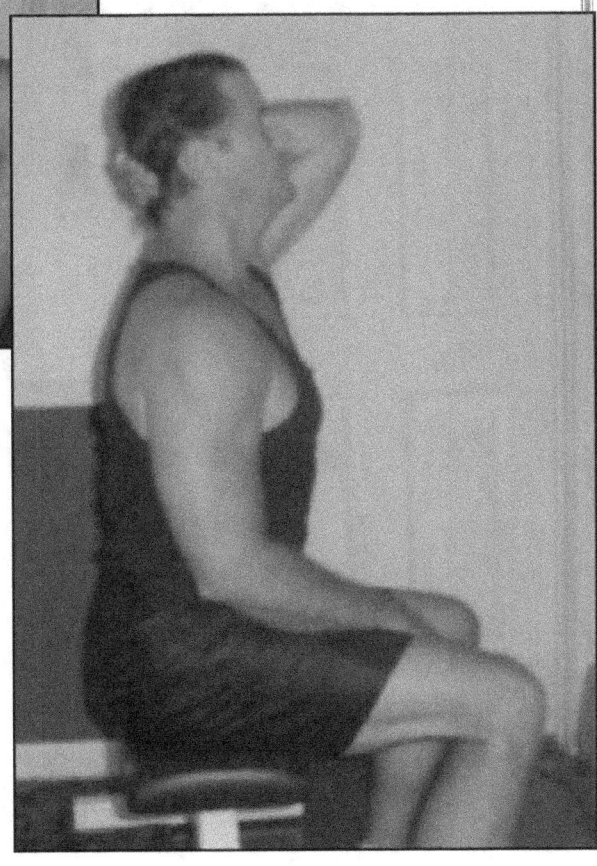

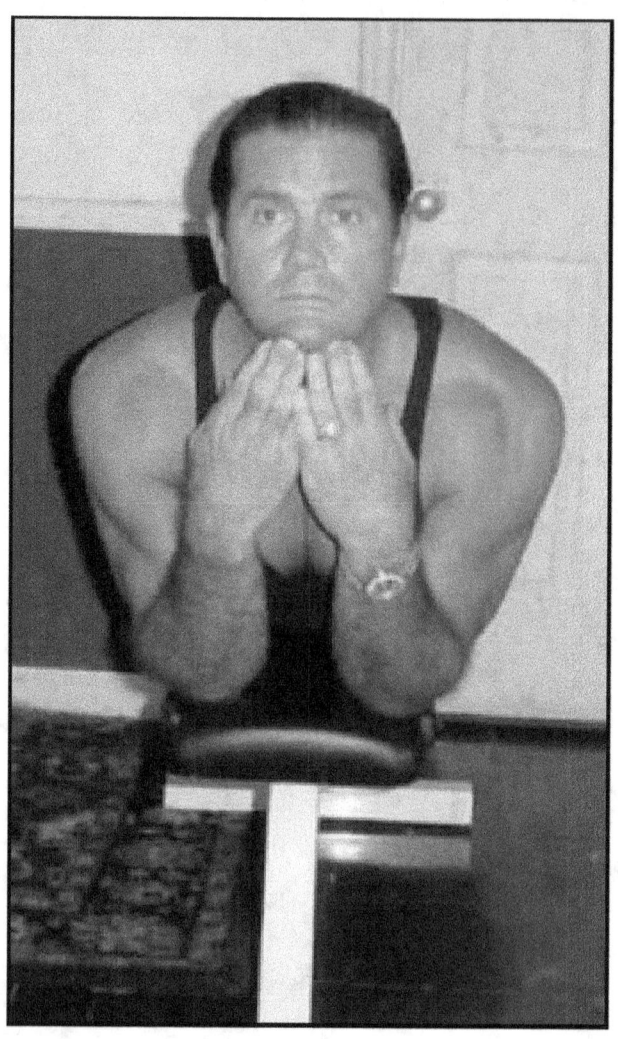

Keep the elbows on the bench and push gently up with the fingers on the chin.
Sit on the bench or chair and place the palm of the hand on the side of the neck,
gently push the head to each side..

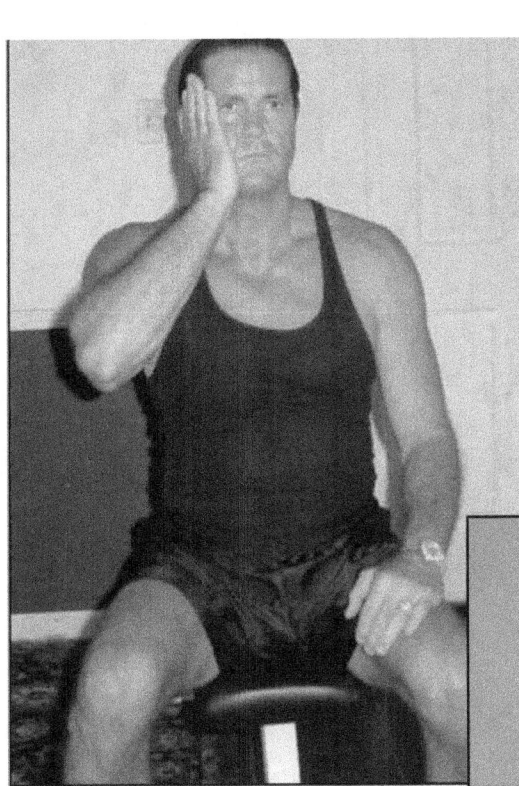

Sit on the bench or chair and place the palm of the hand on the side of the neck, gently push the head to each side..

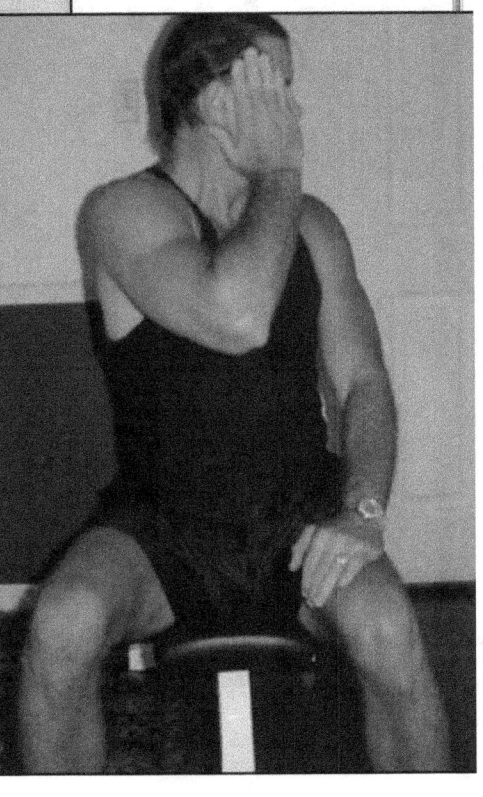

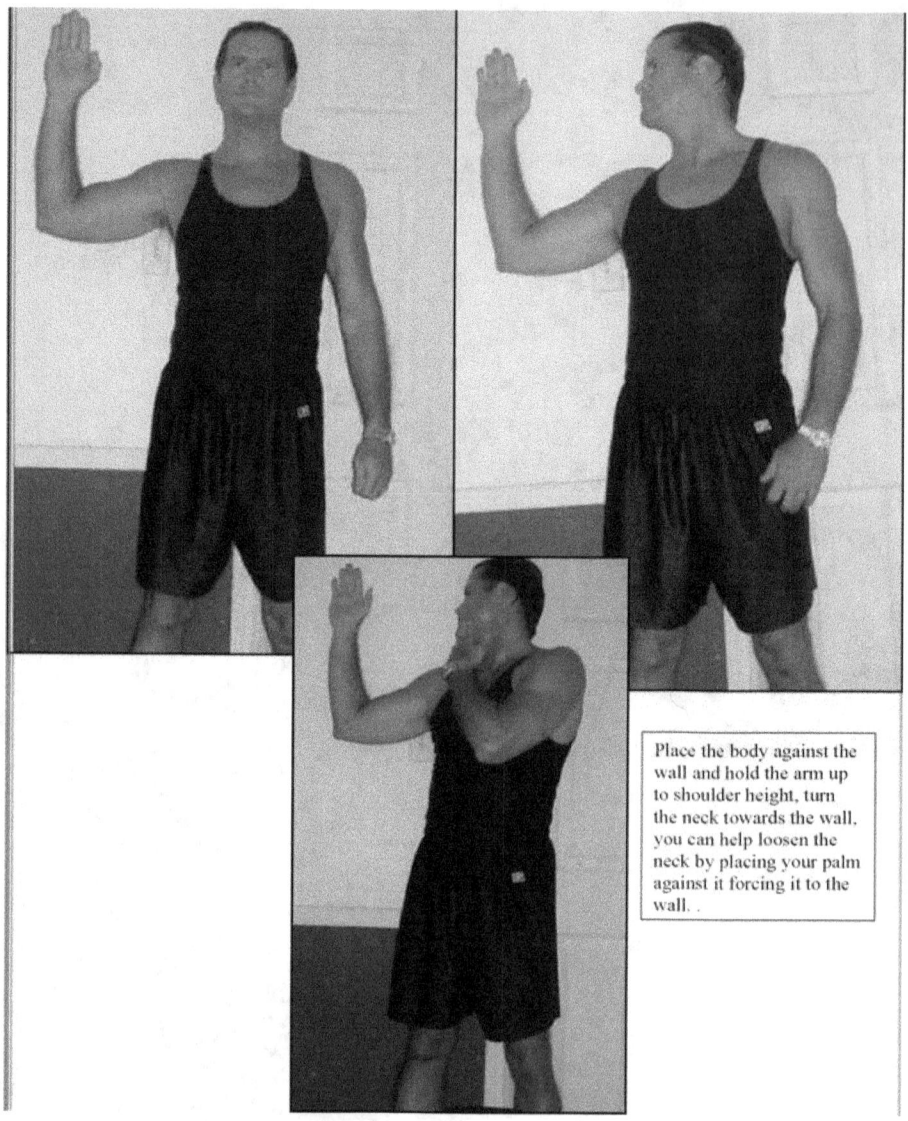

Place the body against the wall and hold the arm up to shoulder height, turn the neck towards the wall, you can help loosen the neck by placing your palm against it forcing it to the wall. .

Place the body against the wall and hold the arm up to shoulder height, turn the neck towards the wall, you can help loosen the neck by placing your palm against it forcing it to the wall. .